COPING SUCCESSFULLY
IRRITABLE BOWEL

ROSEMARY NICOL lives in Somerset, and is married
with four children. As well as the bestselling *Coping
Successfully with Your Irritable Bowel,* she is also the
author of *The Irritable Bowel Diet Book* and *The
Irritable Bowel Stress Book.*

6 666 751 000

Overcoming Common Problems Series

For a full list of titles please contact
Sheldon Press, Marylebone Road, London NW1 4DU

Overcoming Common Problems Series

Overcoming Common Problems Series

Overcoming Common Problems

COPING SUCCESSFULLY
WITH YOUR
IRRITABLE BOWEL

Rosemary Nicol

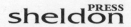

First published in Great Britain in 1989 by
Sheldon Press, SPCK, Marylebone Road, London NW1 4DU

Fourteenth impression 2001

British Library Cataloguing in Publication Data
A catalogue record for this book is available from the British Library
ISBN 0–85969–594–8

Typeset by Deltatype, Ellesmere Port, South Wirral
Printed and bound in Great Britain by
Biddles Ltd, *www.biddles.co.uk*

Contents

Acknowledgements

I would like to acknowledge my gratitude for the invaluable help given to me in the writing of this book. In particular my deepest thanks must go to:

Mr Andrew Gough, Consultant Surgeon, Weston General Hospital, Weston-super-Mare, who wrote the Foreword and gave me so much of his time with help and information; and Dr Enid Smith, General Practitioner, who also answered questions and gave help when I needed it.

In addition I would like to thank the following people who gave help so willingly: Dr Ken Heaton, Reader in Medicine, University of Bristol Department of Medicine; Dr Rosalind Hinton, Member of the British Society of Medical and Dental Hypnosis; Mr Ian MacGregor, Member of the National Institute of Medical Herbalists; Mrs Therese Parsons, Member of the Traditional Acupuncture Society; Mr Steve Sandler, Registered Osteopath, Director of Osteopathic Practice at the British School of Osteopathy; Dr Jeremy Swayne, Homoeopathic Physician, Regional Tutor of the Faculty of Homoeopathic Medicine; and Dr John Hunter, Consultant Physician, Gastro-enterology Research Unit, Addenbrooke's Hospital, Cambridge, and his publishers, Macdonald, for permission to use the exclusion diet, and to reproduce the table on p. 52.

Finally I would like to express my gratitude to my husband, David, for all his help and support; to our children for their tolerance and encouragement, especially our eldest daughter, Katie, who provided me with so much information on food and diet; and to the many people who shared with me their personal experience of living with Irritable Bowel Syndrome.

Foreword

When asked to write an introduction for this book on irritable bowel syndrome (IBS), I was amazed to think that anyone should think it a worthwhile subject for more than a mere leaflet. Only when I took time to reflect did I realize how little information there was available to the sufferer, or indeed, to those who aim to help him or her.

As a gastro-enterologist, I meet people with irritable bowel every working day. They take up a lot of my time, they are worried people and they worry me. The problem with people with IBS is that they do not have a disease, and that is why I have not referred to them as 'patients'. Their disorder is one of gut motility and its symptoms can mimic serious disease. The difficulty with IBS is that it can be a lifelong complaint and although explanation, reassurance, diet and medicine may alleviate the symptoms for a while, in most sufferers they will recur given the right stimulus. That stimulus may be stress, gut infection or food intolerance, or a combination of these factors.

I mentioned that IBS sufferers worry me. This is because traditional Western medicine seeks a pathological cause for symptoms and then aims to cure them. In this case, of course, there is seemingly no pathology and, therefore, no guarantee of cure. To date no one has either devised a test specifically for IBS, or recognized a reproducible characteristic abormality to explain all the symptoms. How then, is it possible to help people with a disorder which appears to have no disease process and which, if apparently successfully treated, may recur? This is where a book such as this one comes in to its own, seeking as it does to explain in a sensible, readable way the state of medical understanding of this condition and to throw light not only on the traditional approach but also on alternative therapies. This seems to me, and I hope to other medical practitioners who may read this book, an entirely creditable exercise. To regard IBS as just a disorder of the bowel is just not tenable these days. It is surely an expression of personality, stress and environment. As medical advisers we must recognize this and give those who come to us for help, the thing that modern hi-tec medicine lacks –*reassurance*. This reassurance and the involvement of the IBS sufferer in his treatment is of vital importance.

1

So if you are unfortunate enough to have IBS I commend this book as a sensible, readable introduction to your understanding of the disorder. I am confident that the sound advice combined in this book will help you (and your doctor) to help yourself.

If you decide that you may have IBS, how should you go about helping yourself?

Assuming your symptoms are typical and that you are otherwise well, I suggest firstly, an examination of your lifestyle. That means a close look at yourself – as you are now, with an assessment of all the things which may tend to put pressure on you. See how you are responding to these pressures and attempt to manoeuvre them in a positive way to your advantage. Look at your diet, your intake of alcohol, your reliance on tablets, such as painkillers and tranquillisers. Be honest with yourself – are all these things not just an indication of your inability to cope with the stresses of life? Make a conscious effort to change your diet to one which contains fresh wholesome foods with the emphasis on fruit, vegetables, cereals and fish and less on meat, dairy products and convenience items. Cut down your alcohol intake. Don't smoke cigarettes, and don't take any tablets or medicines that are not essential and prescribed by your doctor. Take time for yourself each day – to examine what you have done and whether you feel it was worthwhile. Above all, be positive, live your life to the full. You get only one chance at it. Reduce or eliminate those things from your life which affect it, but in a positive way.

I am certain, that if you persevere, then you will be able to control the symptoms of IBS and they will gradually fade into insignificance. Failing this, or if you are not certain that you have IBS or your symptoms are not typical, then ask your doctor for help, he will be sympathetic, quite a proportion of doctors get IBS, too. He won't arrange unpleasant tests, he will talk to you, examine you, give you sound advice, maybe tablets to take for a while, and then will see you again. If you still have symptoms, he may refer you to a hospital specialist, not only because he is unsure, but quite often to reinforce the reassurance.

So I am sure you will see by now, that because you don't have a disease, the best person to help you with your symptoms is you. Quite often the control of these symptoms can help you to find again the purpose of your life.

Andrew Gough MD, FRCS
Surgical Gastro-enterologist

Introduction

You are probably reading this book because you have a condition called Irritable Bowel Syndrome. You may know one or two other people who have it, too. But I expect it isn't something you like to talk about very much – it doesn't often come up in polite conversation, people don't usually compare their irritable bowels over drinks or dinner. The very description of the condition, containing as it does the word 'bowel', tends to keep it rather private.

Yet about one third of the population have had the symptoms of irritable bowel syndrome (IBS) at some time or another, and about 13% of the general population have them regularly. That's a lot of people, and this percentage is common throughout most of the Western world. IBS accounts for about half of all the patients seen by most gastro-enterologists, usually in hospital out-patients departments. So there's a lot of it about; you are not alone.

It would seem reasonable, therefore, to expect IBS to be better known. There are two possible reasons why it isn't. Firstly, we have a natural reluctance to discuss anything to do with the body's nether regions. Most of us were brought up to regard 'bodily functions' as somewhat dirty, faintly disgusting, the subject of crude jokes, and to be kept in their proper place, out of sight and mind. Anything to do with bowels, bowel movements and related matters is definitely not a polite subject in our clean Western culture. Because bowel matters are so little talked about, people often suffer discomfort, distress and embarrassment, in silence. This is a pity, because we all (from the highest in the land to the lowest) have bowel movements, and the way our bowels function is important to our health.

The second reason why irritable bowel syndrome is not generally mentioned is, I suspect, because of its name. To be honest, the words 'irritable' and 'bowel' do not exactly conjure up the sort of image most people would like to have of themselves. If it were called something like 'intestinal motility disorder', or 'functional colon disease', or 'Thingamyjig's syndrome', it might have a better public image. Some medical books do call IBS by different names – 'irritable colon', 'spastic colon', 'mucus colitis', 'spastic colitis', even 'tense tummy' and 'windy bowel' – but none of these has slipped into common usage. So until someone decides on a change

INTRODUCTION

of name, we are stuck with 'irritable bowel syndrome', and I hope
that, by the end of this book, you will have overcome any
embarrassment you might have concerning bodily functions, their
names, and their descriptions.

Rosemary Nicol

1

Who Gets Irritable Bowel Syndrome?

Anybody can get IBS — you, me, Peter at work, Jane next door. Just because friends and work-mates don't talk about it doesn't mean they haven't got it. In fact the chances are that about 13% (that's 1 in 8) of the people you know have it.

When I was asked what I was writing a book about, and I replied 'Irritable Bowel Syndrome', I was amazed at the number of people who said 'I get that'. Often they were people I'd known for a long time; I knew about their families, their jobs, where they were going on holiday, their illnesses, even their politics and religion, but I didn't know about their irritable bowels. Most people keep it very much to themselves.

So, who is most likely to get it? Usually they are people who have recently had a period of stress — the breakup of a relationship, threat of redundancy, money worries, difficulties at home or at work. Also they probably live such busy lives that they don't make time to eat meals in a calm relaxed way.

At one extreme are healthy and robust individuals, who don't go to the doctor about it, and don't feel it upsets their lives in any way. They get is from time to time, but it hardly bothers them. At the other extreme are those for whom IBS is devastating. They daren't move far from a toilet, they feel isolated, panicky, totally lacking in self-confidence. Their social life is ruined, their diet is horribly restricted, and they worry their ill-health may cause them to lose their job. Their tummy becomes the centre of the universe, and they live in fear of the tricks their body may have in store for them. In between, are the great majority, who manage quite well most of the time, but still have to watch what they eat, and find their gut plays them up if they get tense or agitated.

If you don't like the effect IBS has on your life, *take comfort*. There's a lot you can do about it. If the pills and medicines you get from the doctor don't work as well as you'd like, there are plenty of other things you can try. Be prepared to make some changes, to take a new look at yourself, to accept that your health may be in your own hands, and to say 'from today on *I* am going to make me better'.

What exactly is irritable bowel syndrome?

IBS is a disorder of:

(a) *the way in which the contents of the digestive system (i.e. the food you eat) moves through the 30 feet (9 metres) or so of tubing that makes up the large and small intestines* (see the diagram on p. 23, and also Chapter 4 for a definition of all the medical terms you may come across in this book);
(b) *the way these intestines react to various things, particularly diet and stress.*

How and why this happens, and what you can do about it, is the subject of this book.

What are the symptoms of IBS?

For years, patients suffered in silence or went to their doctors with an odd assortment of symptoms which nowadays are recognized as typical of Irritable Bowel Syndrome. These are:

- abdominal pain (i.e. pain in the tummy), usually low down on the left, or possibly centre or right;
- diarrhoea, with or without stomach pain;
- constipation, usually with stomach pain, and small lumpy stools like 'rabbit droppings';
- alternating diarrhoea and constipation, often in an unpredictable and erractic fashion;
- an abdomen that looks or feels bloated and distended;
- feeling 'full of wind';
- passing mucus with the stools, or by itself;
- in addition it generally becomes worse during periods of stress, and may disappear completely at other times.

This particular collection of symptoms is found only in irritable bowel syndrome. Most people with IBS have several of them, particularly pain, together with a tummy that feels distended, and a bowel habit that varies. People with other conditions very seldom have more than two or three of the symptoms.

In addition, if you have IBS, it is quite likely that you will have some of an even longer list of lesser symptoms:

(a) *digestive*
heartburn
nausea
feeling full early in a meal
unpleasant taste in the
   mouth
loss of appetite
regurgitating acid
belching
difficulty in swallowing
rumblings and gurglings
occasional vomiting

(b) *bowel and bladder*
passing urine often
needing to go to the toilet
   urgently
after a bowel movement
   feeling there is more to
   come

(c) *states of mind*
tiredness or lethargy
anxiety
irritation
loss of concentration
mild depression and
   weeping
lack of 'sparkle'

(d) *physical*
back pain
sleeping difficulties
feeling hot behind the eyes
   (like 'flu)
headache, possibly with
   sweating, flushes and
   faintness
reduced sex drive

(e) *extra problems for women*
painful intercourse
painful periods

Is it surprising that, with many of these widely varying complaints, doctors used to think IBS patients were hypochondriacs! But they aren't, and these complaints are now recognized as being extremely common with IBS. Many of them are linked with constipation, so by getting rid of your constipation, you might also get rid of some of the undesirable extras.

In addition, people with IBS are often worried by:

- seeing recognizable food in their stools — this is only because some food has not been properly digested;
- rumblings and gurglings — which are just the digestive process under way;
- passing mucus — this is not a symptom of disease, just of the bowel being over-sensitive;
- the fear of cancer — as you will read more than once in this book, there is no known connection between IBS and bowel cancer.

7

What causes irritable bowel syndrome?

The majority of people can trace their IBS back to:

- an attack of gastro-enteritis — 'holiday tummy' — which may make the intestines over-reactive and sensitive;
- or to a long course of antibiotics, which may alter the delicate balance of natural beneficial bacteria in the body;
- or to an abdominal or pelvic operation;
- or to a stressful time such as divorce, threat of redundancy, unemployment, exams, etc.

Some foods make it worse for some people, but this is probably not the original cause.

Using irritant laxatives too regularly is another major cause — there is a mistaken belief that a daily emptying of the bowels is essential to good health. Also many people with IBS frequently ignore the normal urge to have a bowel movement, thus making matters worse.

From this, you will see that IBS is one of those conditions that people tend to bring upon themselves. If you can eat the sort of diet that does not upset you, if you can avoid laxatives, and if you can learn to reduce stress or at least cope with the stress you have, then you are unlikely to get an irritable bowel.

Before you say to yourself 'well, it's too late now, I've got it', *don't despair*. As various aspects of your life probably triggered it off in the first place, it is likely that, by making some changes in the way you live, you can greatly relieve it, and possibly even be rid of it for ever.

***

I hope that, after reading this chapter, you will be reassured that you are quite normal, like all those other individuals who have IBS. You may have an odd assortment of complaints, but they are all part of this strange syndrome. So read on, and discover how you can live with it, reduce it, and come to terms with it.

2
How Can I Tell?

'When you have eliminated the impossible, whatever remains . . . must be the truth.' Sherlock Holmes in *The Sign of Four*.

Until quite recently, diagnosis of IBS was rather like Sherlock Holmes' famous statement. When presented with a patient with chronic recurring stomach pain, plus assorted other symptoms, the doctor would carry out many and various tests and investigations for numerous diseases, and when thay all proved negative he would pronounce his verdict: 'there's nothing wrong with you', or just possibly 'you haven't got anything particular, therefore you have irritable bowel syndrome'.

This approach was not ideal. For a start, all those consultations and tests were expensive and time-consuming. Then, the doctor's continuing failure to diagnose anything 'real' tended to weaken his patient's confidence in him. The time taken to undergo tests, and wait for results, which then were negative, was dispiriting for the patient and when the final verdict was pronounced, neither doctor nor patient necessarily had total confidence in it. 'He couldn't think what else it might be, so he just said I had irritable bowel syndrome, and I must learn to live with it.'

The problem was that, unlike most diseases, IBS had no real set of clues to aid diagnosis. If you have spotted fever, or mumps, or a peptic ulcer, or almost any gastro-intestinal disease, it can be diagnosed from well-established guidelines. Your doctor can ask questions, examine you, do tests, and come to a firm and confident decision.

IBS is not like that. It is not an organic disease, yet it mimics many other organic diseases; in fact one of the guidelines to a correct diagnosis of IBS is that there is no evidence of any organic disease. The fact that you have certain symptoms, which might well be disease A, B or C, yet you clearly do not have these diseases, is in itself a pointer for the doctor. But it is not just a 'diagnosis of exclusion', that is, exclude everything else and what you have left must be irritable bowel syndrome. There are now several clearly defined symptoms which, if you have them, mean you have IBS.

Before we look at these, it is worth looking at the problems of diagnosis from your doctor's viewpoint. His patient has the sort of symptoms that could, on first appearance, be any one of a number of diseases. The persistent pain, the distended abdomen, the constipation and diarrhoea, and the assorted other symptoms (headache, tiredness, nausea, back pain) could all be caused by something that he mustn't overlook. In addition, his patient may be thinking all this too, and be fearful that she has cancer or some serious bowel disorder. It is obviously most important that he does not miss anything.

Because of this, many doctors used to be tempted to try a 'shotgun' approach, that is, arrange tests and investigations for every conceivable disorder, and hope that one of them shows up something. This can reflect the doctor's uncertainty, and the more tests that are carried out the more anxious the patient is likely to become, and this anxiety can undermine the relationship between them.

Fortunately, this is not now necessary. Thanks to a lot of research that has been done on the irritable bowel, there are at last clear guidelines for diagnosis. If you, the sufferer, are aware of these, it is likely that when your doctor tells you that you have irritable bowel syndrome, you will believe him. And having believed him you will be in a good position to work towards coping with it.

IBS is not a physical disease: it is a disorder in the way part of the digestive system functions. It is unlikely to get much worse, but for some people it may never get completely better. Once you can accept that, and learn how to control it, you will find it much easier to live with. Rest assured that there is no known link between IBS and cancer of the digestive system, nor is it life-threatening. It may cause you pain, inconvenience, and even distress, but it will not kill you.

And under the following circumstances, you can be confident that what you have got is irritable bowel syndrome, and not anything else:

1. The more of the following symptoms that you have, the more likely it is that you have IBS, as people with other disorders very seldom have more than two or three of them at most (see Chapter 4 for any medical terms you don't understand):
- pain which improves by having a bowel movement
- loose stools when the pain starts
- more frequent stools when the pain starts

- pellety stools 'like rabbit droppings'
- alternating diarrhoea and constipation
- bloating and distension of the abdomen, often with wind
- the feeling, after a bowel movement, that there is more to come
- passing mucus with the stools

2. If you have had a sigmoidoscopy, barium enema, blood tests, and a physical examination of the back passage, and they all prove normal. (If you are under 40, and other tests are normal, your doctor may decide the sigmoidoscopy and barium enema are not necessary). You will read more about these tests in Chapter 6.

3. If you have no serious loss of weight, if you do not pass blood in the stools, and if you have had this condition for quite a long time (say, two years or more).

4. If your doctor has taken a detailed medical history from you, and the previous three conditions apply, and he now tells you 'you have irritable bowel syndrome', then it is highly likely that you can have complete confidence in his diagnosis.

From this, you will see that a positive diagnosis of IBS does involve a doctor; you cannot be totally confident without his help. For this reason, if you think you may have IBS (or any other medical condition), it is important to get it correctly diagnosed by a doctor. Don't rush straight into self-treatment — you may overlook something serious.

Here, too, are some extra thoughts to reassure you about the diagnosis. If the pain is colicky or spasmodic (as it usually is with IBS), that probably means it is coming from somewhere where things are moving, i.e. a tube. This narrows the possible area down to the intestines. If you are under about 40, it is most unlikely that you have cancer of the colon or rectum. If you are over 40, the doctor will probably check for these, and if the tests are negative believe him. As I have mentioned before, there is no documented mortality or serious disease connected with IBS.

So, IBS *is*:
- a problem of how your insides work;
- a disorder in the way food moves through the intestines;
- aggravated by stress and, for some people, the wrong diet;
- a condition which comes and goes;

- tiresome;
- surprisingly common.

And IBS *is not*:
- cancer, or related in any way to cancer;
- inflammatory bowel disease, ulcerative colitis, Crohn's disease, or any other serious bowel disease;
- an organic disease;
- life-threatening;
- suffered only by neurotics and hypochondriacs;
- something else.

As so many people with IBS fear they may have cancer, it is obviously important for you to feel reassured that you have not. Bowel cancer kills more people in the Western world than any other cancer except lung cancer, yet has a good cure rate if it is detected early. For this reason, if you are seriously worried, get it checked as soon as possible by a doctor – if you do have cancer you will have greatly increased your chances of recovery; if the doctor says that you have irritable bowel syndrome, believe him, and read the rest of this book.

3

'It's all in your mind, Mrs Jones'

But it isn't, is it? It's right there, in your insides, only other people don't really believe you. 'If only you'd pull yourself together, stop worrying about it and join an evening class, it would all disappear.' And everybody (your doctor, your family and friends, your boss) could have a quiet life.

While researching this book, I read several dozen papers in highly reputable medical journals, and so often the same words kept cropping up: neurotic, aggressive, anxious, depressed, obsessive. There is little doubt that many doctors still regard this as the classic description of someone with an irritable bowel, so they tell their patients that it's due to their 'nerves', that the symptoms are largely imaginary, or at least greatly exaggerated, and they prescribe tranquillisers.

Now *you* know this is unjust, but why do some doctors not see that? To be fair to them, there is little doubt that many people with irritable bowel syndrome *who visit their doctor* tend to have more general complaints than the population at large. They are more likely to see the doctor for a cold or 'flu than to treat it themselves. They are more likely to have days off work, headaches, and sleep difficulties. They have more problems at work, anxiety over their children or their parents, concern about their marriage, and they worry more about small problems than most people do. In general, these particular people are more likely to visit the doctor and rely on him than to take responsibility for their own health. They also have a greater fear of cancer and other serious diseases, and the anxiety that this generates may aggravate their IBS symptoms.

Yet doctors are seeing a self-selected group: those who have decided to visit the doctor. This group is not typical. The vast majority of people with IBS do not see a doctor at all; they don't regard their condition as serious or abnormal in any way, and they are in other respects robust, healthy people. They seek no advice, and do not bring their bowels to the doctor's attention.

So people who *do* see the doctor about their irritable bowel are a small group, not typical of the majority. And those who progress beyond the doctor, to the hospital specialist, and still further to volunteer in IBS research and drug trials (which are then written up

13

in learned journals) are a smaller group still. Many researchers make the mistake of assuming that the people they see in hospital surveys are typical, when they are not, and then of assuming that what they have discovered in a small, self-selected and untypical group applies to everyone else with IBS, even to those who seek no medical help. Although people with IBS make up about half the patients seen by most gastro-enterologists, it is quite unfair to label everyone with this condition as neurotic and over-anxious. Thirteen per cent of apparently healthy people in Britain have IBS, yet the great majority seek help only from their general practitioners or not at all.

So let us now look at why some doctors put these rather unattractive labels on so many people. Our fictitious Mrs Jones visits the doctor again. She's already been many times before, usually about a pain in her abdomen, though she also has headaches, wind, sleeping problems, and she does seem rather anxious about things in general. (Although I have chosen a woman as our typical doctor's patient, the condition is spread fairly evenly between men and women. It is, however, the women who are most likely to see their doctors. I wonder why this is? Also, by making the patient female, I can distinguish her from a male doctor; of course, the situation may commonly be reversed – a male patient seeing a female doctor.)

The doctor's heart sinks when he sees her. 'What is it this time?' he thinks to himself. He has prescribed a variety of medicines for her (which don't appear to have had much success), he's examined her (and found nothing wrong), he's referred her to the specialist (who also found nothing wrong), and the specialist arranged for her to have tests (which all proved normal). If there is nothing wrong with her then surely she must be imagining things? He has a waiting room full of people with real complaints that respond to his treatments and tests in the way he expects them to, and, quite honestly, he is beginning to lose patience with Mrs Jones. So he tells her she has irritable bowel syndrome (that should keep her happy), says she must stop worrying about things, and prescribes some tranquillisers to calm her down, plus some anti-spasmodics and a bulk laxative.

Looking at it objectively, the doctor's viewpoint does not seem *totally* unreasonable, does it?

From Mrs Jones's viewpoint, however, things look rather different. She has had a pain in her tummy for quite a long time, together with bowel habits that are quite variable – sometimes constipation, sometimes diarrhoea. She feels full of wind, too, but her most worrying problem is the tummy ache. The trouble is that nothing seems to make it better. She's tried indigestion tablets, laxatives, and a whole range of painkillers, and still it never goes away for long. In Mrs Jones's mind, a pain that never really gets better, and that doesn't respond to painkillers, is worrying. Why doesn't it get better? Could it be something serious, like cancer? She sees her doctor, who prescribes medicines which don't work. She gets more worried. The doctor sends her to hospital for various tests, and they all conclude that there is nothing wrong with her. But there *must* be something wrong. Why does she keep getting this pain, and such topsy-turvey bowel habits? Is the doctor keeping some dreadful truth from her? Should she perhaps find a different doctor?

Poor Mrs Jones. To have symptoms which distress her and reduce the quality of her life is bad enough. Worse still to find that no one seems to know what causes them. And the last straw to realize that her doctor thinks she's making it all up.

I know that I am being unfair to a great many doctors who *do* know about IBS. Although they realize it can be related to stress, they also know it has clearly recognized physical causes, they do not dismiss it as 'all in the mind', and they take time to explain the condition to their patients, to reassure them, and to prescribe treatments (such as a high-fibre diet and anti-spasmodic medicines) that will almost certainly work.

Even so, they are still treating the symptoms, without always taking the time to discover the main underlying causes – stress and, in some cases, diet. If they could help their patients to identify the stressful events in their lives, to learn how to reduce them, or at least find them less stressful, and to eat foods that do not disagree with them, it is highly likely that IBS would take up less of their time. But how many busy doctors can find time to teach relaxation, and work out individual diet sheets? And should that really be part of a doctor's job?

Recognizing that IBS is *not* 'all in the mind' is half the battle. There are indeed physical causes, and, to be fair to your unsympathetic doctor, many of these physical causes are aggravated by states of mind.

You will almost certainly have noticed that, when you are slightly nervous or anxious about anything, you get 'butterflies' in your tummy; you may also need to go to the toilet more often, and you may possibly not feel much like eating. These are quite normal reactions, and they occur because there are direct nerve pathways between the brain and the gut. Quite simply, how your mind feels affects how your stomach behaves, and conversely, if your stomach is all churned up your mind will be churned up, too. There is nothing unusual about this.

When you are under stress of any kind, your stomach will produce more hydrochloric acid, which causes your bowel to contract more vigorously than normal.

If you have IBS you may also have other physical conditions which trigger your disturbed gut:

- You probably have some abnormality in the way the muscle of your large intestine propels its contents, which is either inherited or caused by previous gastro-intestinal infections. Because of this, your muscles are likely to contract more vigorously than normal, causing spasm and pain.
- The muscles of your intestines may be extra-sensitive.
- You may produce more mucus than usual.
- Gastro-enteritis or a long course of antibiotics can cause changes to take place in the useful bacteria that live in the gut and that help in the normal process of digestion.
- Different foods cause the intestines to produce different chemicals, and your gut may over-react to some of these chemicals.
- Pain is not measurable scientifically – we all feel it at different levels. What is mild discomfort to one person may be severe pain to another. Perhaps some people with IBS feel pain at particularly low levels.
- Almost certainly, the nature of your bowel means that you feel more pain than usual when the lower bowel (the rectum) is full, as in constipation. This fullness in the bowel may produce pain in the most unlikely places – the back, shoulders, thigh, and the area in front of the anus.
- If you have diarrhoea as the main symptom you may have an 'incompetent sigmoid colon', which means that the last part of the colon does not work as well as it should, and allows sloppy contents to descend into the rectum before all the water has been absorbed.

These physical causes are real and recognizable, and are not 'in the mind'.

However, this doesn't mean that you can't do anything about them. You can. Firstly, if your bowel muscles contract more vigorously than usual, it is important to make sure the contents of the bowel are soft and bulky, not hard and small. And if your lower bowel feels pain when it is full more than other people's bowels do, then try not to get your bowel over-full. The answer to both these is to eat a diet that is full of fibre, and to make sure you do not become constipated (see Chapters 8 and 9).

If you get a lot of diarrhoea, this may well be due to stress, but it could also be due to a clear physical cause: perhaps your body does not produce enough of the enzyme lactase to digest the milk products you eat. If you are referred to a gastro-enterologist, this is one of the tests he may arrange for you. If it turns out that you do have some intolerance to milk products, then you would be well advised to take less of them.

Again, the solution to so many digestive problems is in your own hands and not necessarily to take medicines. Ask yourself not 'what shall I take for this', but 'what can I do about this'.

Finally, let us suppose that your IBS does cause you to be difficult to live with at times. Is this really surprising? The very nature of IBS can reduce your self-confidence. Having continuing pain will obviously affect the quality of your life. Always having to watch what you eat can play havoc with your social life, and the constant need to be near a toilet does nothing for your self-esteem. Having chronic symptoms which the doctor seems unable to diagnose is worrying. The need to discuss bowels and bowel movements is distasteful to many people, as is the thought of being examined in that area of the body. And if your family, your friends, your boss, and even your doctor are not particularly sympathetic, is it surprising you may get anxious, depressed, moody, and yes, maybe even neurotic or obsessive about it?

Take comfort. There is a great deal you can do to help yourself. By the time you have finished this book, you will have a good idea how you can keep your irritable bowel very much under control.

4
What Are They Talking About?

You've waited three months for an appointment to see the specialist; now you've waited for an hour in the out-patients department. At last: 'Mrs Jones, Room 7, please'. In Room 7 are two doctors and a nurse.

'Good morning, come in. It's Mrs Jones, isn't it? What's your problem? Yes, yes, yes, I see, I see.'

From then on you might as well not be there. Words and phrases you've never heard before are tossed around from one doctor to the other – post-prandial pain (does that mean pain in my tummy?), rectal dissatisfaction (I'm not particularly dissatisfied), irritable bowel (me? irritable?), motility, intestinal transit, we'll do a sigmoidoscopy (a what?) and a barium enema (I don't like the sound of *that*).

'Thank you Mrs Jones, we'll arrange some tests for you. Goodbye, next please.'

Well, what was all *that* about? They were talking about you, but did you understand what they were saying?

So many of us wait passively for *them* to do things to us – *they* make appointments for us, *they* ask the questions (*we* don't), *they* do the tests, *they* carry out the treatment.

But it's *your* body. You've lived with it all your life, fed it, washed it, clothed it, exercised it, cared for it. The more you understand how it works, what it can do for you, why it goes wrong and, most important, how *you* can help put it right, the more you will be in control of your own health.

So this chapter and the next will help you to understand what is going on, in the belief that by controlling your own body you have a much greater chance of making yourself well.

This chapter is about the many words and phrases you may hear doctors using about irritable bowel syndrome. If the words wash over your head you are not in a position to help your own recovery; if you understand what they mean you are half way there. You can also use the pages which follow to check on the meaning of words you may not understand that occur in this book. The next chapter describes the digestive system.

Abdominal: anything to do with the abdomen, or tummy.

Abdominal distension: your tummy feels, or looks, bloated and full.

Anti-spasmodic: a drug used to reduce spasm and to loosen tight muscles.

Anal spasm: when the muscle of the *anus* goes into sudden contraction.

Anus: the circular band of muscle at the lower end of the *rectum*.

Barium enema: a test that can be carried out (see Chapter 6).

Bowel: the area you may vaguely think of as your 'insides'. It consists of the small intestine (which is about 20 ft (6 metres) long), and the large intestine (which is about 5 ft (150cm) long), and covers the area from the bottom of your ribs downwards (see Chapter 5).

Bulking agents: usually a form of fibre (such as Fybogel or Isogel or Regulan) given to bulk out the stools and make them soft and easier to pass.

Call to stool: the urge to go to the toilet and have a bowel movement.

Colic: severe pain in the *abdomen*, caused by *spasm* of the muscles.

Colon: the main part of the large intestine (see Chapter 5).

Constipation: straining to pass stools.

Defecation: the act of emptying the bowels; having a bowel movement.

Diarrhoea: passing watery motions.

Dyspareunia: pain during sexual intercourse.

Enzyme: a substance that, during digestion, breaks down what we eat into a form in which it can be used by the body. (In IBS some people do not produce enough of the enzyme *lactase* which breaks down the sugars in dairy products.)

Faeces (pronounced 'fee-sees'): the waste that you pass when you have a bowel movement. Also known as 'stools', or 'motions'.

Familial: anything which runs in the family.

Flatulence: feeling full of wind.

Flatus: wind, the gas that builds up in your gut.

Fibre: substance found in the cell wall of plants, which is not absorbed and digested by the human gut.

Functional: a condition that has no known physical cause, and so is assumed to be caused by the personality or the environment.

Gastro-intestinal: concerning that part of your body which deals with the digestion of food.

Idiopathic: used to describe a condition which has no apparent cause.

Intermittent pain: a pain that is not constant, but occurs from time to time.

Intestinal transit: the movement of food through your digestive system.

Intolerance (to food): certain foods disagree with you, and possibly make your IBS worse (see Chapter 12).

Lactase: an enzyme that breaks down *lactose* during the process of digestion. Some people do not have enough of this enzyme in their bodies, so cannot digest dairy products properly.

Lactose: a sugar that occurs naturally in milk, and which can make IBS worse in some people.

Laxative: something you take to stop constipation.

Micturition: the act of emptying the bladder, passing water.

Motility: the speed with which food passes through your system, from the time you put it in your mouth until you pass it out as a bowel movement.

Mucus: a slimy substance, sometimes passed with a bowel movement in IBS, or even by itself.

Nausea: feeling sick.

Organic disease: something wrong with one or more of your internal organs. Many IBS sufferers fear they have an organic disease such as cancer or ulcerative colitis, whereas IBS is more a problem concerning how your digestive system is working.

Over-reactive: the term applied to a gut which reacts more than normal to stimuli such as certain foods, distension, stress, etc.

Physiological: to do with the normal working of the body.

Post-prandial pain: a pain, usually in the tummy, that comes on after meals.

Prognosis: how the doctor thinks the condition will progress, how long it will last, what will happen next.

Purgative: see *laxative*.

Rectal dissatisfaction: the feeling, after you have completed a bowel movement, that you haven't finished yet, that there is still more to come.

Rectum: the last part of the large intestine, where waste matter is stored before finally being passed out of your body through the *anus* (the back passage).

Refractory: used to describe something that doesn't respond well to treatment.

Sigmoidoscopy: a test that can be carried out (see Chapter 6).

Spasm: sudden contraction of the muscles.

Spastic: being in a state of *spasm*. Much of the pain of IBS is because muscles are in spasm, and tighten up, and the pain comes in waves; that is why doctors often prescribe *anti-spasmodic drugs*.

Syndrome: a collection of symptoms all together.

Urinary frequency: wanting to empty the bladder often.

Vomiting: actually being sick.

Now that you understand the meaning of the words doctors may use about irritable bowel syndrome, you may be interested to know more about the area of your body that all this applies to – the digestive system.

5
The Digestive System

The food you eat is not much use to your body in the form of fish and chips, lentils, roast beef, apples, bread, cream cakes, yoghurt, or anything else you put in your mouth. For all these complicated things to be useful, they must be broken down into simple substances that your body can make use of. This is the process of digestion. Proteins become amino acids, to build muscles, hair, nails, skin, kidney and liver cells, and bone marrow. Fats are absorbed, and stored as a source of future energy. They also provide body fat for warmth, and to protect bones and organs. Carbohydrates become sugars to provide energy for instant use. Vitamins and minerals are extracted, many of which are important in maintaining good health.

To complete the process of digestion, the food travels along about 40 feet (12 metres) of tubing, is ground up, churned about, dissolved, broken down, acted upon by chemicals, has water drawn from it, and finally leaves your body a day or two later (see the diagram on page 23).

When you put food in your mouth, your teeth cut and grind it. Saliva helps the teeth to break it down, and also makes it slippery in order to enable it to slide down the *oesophagus* (or gullet). It is squeezed down the oesophagus by *peristalsis*, a process involving alternate waves of muscular relaxation and contraction, which occurs at most stages of digestion, including in the bowel, as we will see later.

From there the food enters the stomach. To most people's surprise, the stomach is not in the middle of the tummy, but behind the ribs; it is a muscular bag which prepares food for absorption into the bloodstream, and in it the food is churned around like in a food mixer for about 2–4 hours. When enzymes and acids have worked on it, the food leaves the stomach looking rather like a thick soup.

The rest of the digestive process takes place in about 30 feet (9 metres) of tubing called the bowel, and so is of interest to you if you have IBS.

The first 20 feet (6 metres) or so of bowel is the *small intestine* – called 'small' because the tube is only just over 1 inch (3 cm) in diameter. It is all coiled up in the central part of the tummy,

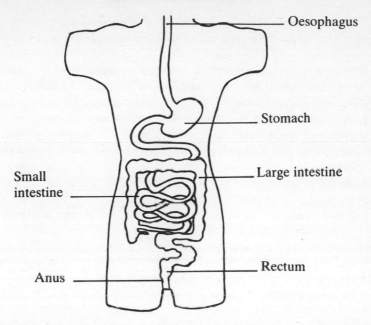

Oesophagus

Stomach

Small intestine

Large intestine

Anus

Rectum

approximately behind the umbilicus (belly button). For several hours digestive juices act on it until it is liquid enough to be absorbed through the walls of the small intestine and into the bloodstream so it can be carried away all around the body, to be used for making, building and repairing.

For the food that is still left, the next stop is the *large intestine*, also known as the *colon*. The changeover point between small and large intestine is low down on the right-hand side of your tummy, and here the large intestine starts. It is about 2½ inches (6 cm) wide and about 5 feet (150 cm) long, and wrinkled like a concertina. It passes up the right hand side, across the middle of your tummy about level with your belly button, and down the left hand side, and this is the direction that the food travels in the large intestine, taking about 1–3 days. Here the last stages of digestion are completed, as water from the semi-liquid mass is absorbed back into the body, and the waste material that is left is stored temporarily until there is enough for it to be passed out of the body.

By the time it reaches the end of the large intestine and passes into the rectum at the bottom left hand side of the tummy, it is quite compact, fairly dry, and brown. Glands produce mucus, which forms a protective coating for the faeces, and makes it easier for it to pass out of the anus. The anus is a strong band of muscle which opens to allow waste material to leave, and then closes tightly afterwards.

Food is moved along the large intestine by muscular waves, called 'peristalsis'. These waves are stimulated by three conditions:

- A large volume of waste material being present inside you.
- By filling the stomach with another meal which causes signals to be sent to the brain to 'open bowels and make room for the next lot'.
- By taking exercise.

It is the nature of peristalsis that causes some of the symptoms of IBS, and which will be discussed later on.

6
Medical Investigations and Treatments

> It is a good rule of thumb that if many treatments are in use for the same disease, it is because there is no real treatment known for that disease. Peter Parish, *Medicines: A Guide for Everybody*.

In the past, indeed until quite recently, people with IBS had appendices removed, intensive abdominal investigations, major gynaecological operations, numerous X-rays, and would take a whole range of pills and potions to rid them of the strange collection of symptoms we now recognize as irritable bowel syndrome. Not surprisingly, these drastic measures were not usually very successful as doctors were seldom treating the real cause of the problem. Luckily, things are different now.

The first thing your doctor will want to do is make a correct diagnosis, to make sure that what you have really is IBS, and not something else (see Chapter 2). Having done that, he will recommend treatment.

Even if you decide that you want to treat your condition yourself, or you want to receive treatment from a practitioner of alternative medicine (see Chapters 20 and 21), it really is most important that first of all you get a correct diagnosis from a medically qualified doctor. That way you can be sure that you are treating the right thing, and that nothing serious is being overlooked.

The first part of this chapter deals with the more usual investigations you may have. They may take place in your doctor's surgery, or in a hospital outpatients department. It is unlikely you would have to stay in hospital as an inpatient. Typically, in the past, patients would have a whole range of tests, and when they all proved normal the verdict would be irritable bowel syndrome. Now, if you are under about 40, the doctor may feel confident to make the diagnosis on your medical history and a brief physical examination alone, and without arranging any tests.

The second part of the chapter covers the drugs and other treatments the doctor may recommend, having reached his diagnosis. Alternative and self-help methods are discussed in later chapters.

First, the doctor will ask you a series of questions. The answers to

25

these questions will often enable the doctor to decide whether you have IBS without the need to subject you to lots of tests.

He will probably ask you:

- When did you first start getting these symptoms?
- Did anything specific trigger it off?
- How often does it occur?
- Where exactly is the pain?
- Have you had diarrhoea and/or constipation before?
- Do your bowel habits change?
- Have they recently changed?
- Have you lost weight recently?
- Does your tummy look or feel bloated and distended?
- Do you pass mucus with a bowel movement, or even on its own?
- Have you ever had bleeding from the back passage?
- Have you recently had a bout of gastro-enteritis ('holiday tummy')?
- Did you get tummy ache as a child?
- Did any of your family have these symptoms?
- Does it become worse when you are tense, anxious or stressed?
- Or when you eat particular foods?
- Can you do anything to make the symptoms better or worse?
- Do any of your family have an intolerance to dairy products, or to wheat products, and how much of these do you eat?

Then, depending on the answers, and on your age, he may suggest some physical tests. He may do some of them himself, or refer you to a specialist at a hospital. If you are under about 40, he may want to check for a peptic ulcer, for gall bladder disease, ulcerative colitis, and Crohn's disease. If you are over about 40, he will also want to be sure there is no sign of malignancy (cancer) in the bowel.

Because of the nature of IBS, it is not at present possible to do a single test and say 'this test is positive, therefore you have irritable bowel syndrome'. So, in some cases the doctor will want to do one or two investigations to rule out the diseases that IBS mimics before he can come to a firm conclusion that you and he can have confidence in.

The first test will almost certainly be a *rectal examination*, that is, an examination of the rectum. He will probably ask you to take off your clothes below the waist, to lie on the examination couch on your left side, and bend your legs up slightly. After putting on thin rubber gloves, he will insert one finger into the rectum, and feel around inside. This simple test will be able to tell him about the condition of your rectum. It will probably be a bit uncomfortable, and you may feel embarrassed, but don't forget that he does this kind of thing every day, and it is all quite run of the mill to him. A good doctor will recognize your embarrassment, and will do all he can to put you at ease.

The three most likely investigations for IBS are: blood tests, a sigmoidoscopy, and a barium enema.

Most people have had *blood tests* from time to time. A small area of skin, usually in the arm, is cleaned with an alcohol swab. A fine needle is inserted into a vein, and a small quantity of blood is drawn out into a syringe. This sample will be sent away to be checked for generalized infection, anaemia, and the state of the liver and kidneys.

A *sigmoidoscopy* is an investigation to test for disease in the rectum and lower colon. You will be asked to lie in the same position as for the rectal examination. The doctor will insert into the rectum one end of an instrument called a 'sigmoidoscope', which is a tube just under an inch (about 2 cm) in diameter and 12 inches (30 cm) long, with a light at the end. By shining the light right up into the rectum he will be able to see clearly the condition of the rectum and the lower end of the colon. Any growths (cancerous or non-cancerous) will be visible to him, as will any other abnormal condition, such as inflammation. This examination, as you can imagine, can be quite uncomfortable, and for some people may be rather painful. But most people who have it feel reassured that the whole area has been thoroughly looked at. If, having looked, the doctor now says that you do not have any inflammation, or cancer of the rectum, you will probably feel greatly relieved. A sigmoidoscopy has one other benefit: the process of inserting the tube into the rectum causes the rectum to become distended, and often reproduces exactly the sort of pain you get with IBS. Many people are reassured to make the connection between a distended rectum and the pain of IBS, and therefore feel more motivated to take steps to avoid constipation.

A *barium enema* helps to check for organic disease of the whole colon, and can also provide evidence of an 'irritable' colon. For a barium enema to be successful, you will need to have an almost empty digestive system. So you will be asked not to eat anything for

27

several hours beforehand. Back in the X-ray department, a tube will be inserted into the rectum, and a small quantity of thick white liquid passed through it. So that the liquid can reach every part of the bowel, this procedure may be carried out on a table that allows you to be tilted slightly in different positions. The tube is then withdrawn. The white liquid will show up brightly on the X-ray, and any problems or irregularities over the entire length of the large intestine will be clearly visible. If you have a 'spastic' or 'irritable' colon, this will also show up. After the X-ray you will eliminate the white liquid as if it were a very runny bowel movement plus wind.

Some hospitals have a slightly different procedure: you will be asked to eat nothing after midnight, and to take a laxative at bedtime. Next day you may have a simple X-ray of the abdominal area, and after that undergo the same procedure for filling up the intestine with a thick white liquid. This is then X-rayed. You may then be asked to empty your bowel for the whole area to be X-rayed again.

If diarrhoea is your main symptom you may also have tests for lactose intolerance (see Chapter 6), and possibly a biopsy of the small intestine. For the biopsy, you swallow a small metal capsule attached to a suction tube; when the capsule reaches the right part of the bowel, the doctor will apply suction to the tube, and a tiny piece from the wall of the bowel will be sucked into the capsule and removed for examination.

Just a word here about tests in general. Most people are pleased to have tests to get reassurance that they have nothing seriously wrong with them; when the results are normal they consider that the end of the matter. However, there is a small group of people who like having tests, who like having a hospital appointment to keep, who even like having operations. Are you one of these? If so, recognize it in yourself, and realize that being like this may cause you to receive less sympathy than you feel you deserve from your doctor, your family and your friends.

In the past (and unfortunately even now occasionally), many doctors would say something like 'we have done tests, and there is nothing wrong with you', and leave it at that. If you still complained of stomach pain, or changeable bowel habits, or a distended tummy, he would probably dismiss this as the complaints of a hypochondriac, prescribe tranquillisers, and hope you would go away. After all, as he said, 'tests prove that there is nothing wrong with you'.

Today, particularly if you have a kind and caring doctor, he may say 'we will do some tests just to check that you haven't got disease A, B, or C, and I expect the tests will be normal'. So, when they are normal, this is just what you and he expect. And he will probably go on to explain that you have irritable bowel syndrome, and to outline what it is, what it is not, how he can help you, and also how you can help yourself.

IBS cannot be helped by having an operation, but there are several drugs that are very effective. The most common ones are:

- *Anti-spasmodics* to make the bowel muscle relax and relieve the colicky spasm that causes so much pain. They appear to have no serious side-effects, though they may impair driving ability, or affect your blood pressure.
- *Bulk laxatives*, usually based on the fibre ispaghula. As explained in Chapter 10, they make the stools soft, bulky and easy to pass. They, too, appear to have no side-effects.
- *Mild anti-depressants* to relieve the stress and anxiety that is probably making your irritable bowel worse. But they usually have side-effects, and it is not in your best interests to continue the long-term use of drugs that affect your mind. In any case, used by themselves, and without anti-spasmodics or bulk laxatives, they don't appear to give much improvement to IBS.

Where wind is a problem, peppermint oil capsules are often effective. You can obtain much the same effect yourself by sipping a few drops of peppermint essence in a small glass of warm water, or by sucking sweets containing oil of peppermint (see also Chapter 7).

For diarrhoea, you may be prescribed substances such as codeine phosphate or loperamide (see also Chapter 11).

For constipation the most effective drugs are the bulk laxatives; you will probably be advised to eat more fibre in your diet (see Chapter 8, 9 and 10). Don't be tempted to take laxatives that you buy over the counter. Unless used extremely rarely, they can make IBS worse.

For other ways to reduce stomach pain see Chapter 7.

In treating IBS, many doctors prescribe three types of drug (an anti-spasmodic plus a bulk laxative plus a mild short-term anti-depressant). This is usually quite effective, particularly over a short period. But as IBS is often a long-term disorder, drugs cannot really be the right answer permanently. If you can accept that what you eat, how you live, and how you view life will probably have more effect on your bowel than anything else, you are already half-way to coping with it.

It should really be your aim to take drugs for as short a time as possible. Once the bulk laxatives have given you a soft unformed motion every day for two weeks, see if you can keep this up by diet alone. For most people it should be possible.

When you are confident that the anti-spasmodic will reduce your stomach pain, take a fresh look at the tension in you that is causing your bowel muscles to seize up. Then you will become less dependent on drugs. After all, if you see drugs as the only way of getting relief, you may feel a sense of helplessness and dependence on them; when you realize you can improve your condition for yourself, this will lift up your spirits as you take control of your own health.

From Chapter 7 onwards you will find many ideas on how you can help yourself. There is no suggestion in this book that you will find a permanent life-long cure, because for many people this just will not happen. The longer you have had IBS the harder it is to be rid of it completely. But there is no doubt at all that by tackling it in the right way, you should be able to live more happily with it.

Hopefully, once your IBS has been diagnosed, and treatment (conventional or alternative) started, you will not need to visit your doctor as often as you might have done before. But there are other causes of abdominal pain, and even IBS sufferers can get appendicitis, peptic ulcers and heart trouble. Also, although IBS doesn't cause cancer, it doesn't prevent it either. So there are a few symptoms which, if they should occur, you must not ignore:

- blood in the stools, or in urine;
- vomiting blood;
- very severe abdominal pain;
- 'indigestion'-type pain which persists for more than a day or two;
- excessive thirst;
- unexplained loss of weight or appetite;
- unexplained change in bowel habits that lasts for a month or more and which causes disruption to your life;
- unexplained increase in the size of your stomach;
- IBS symptoms which change or get noticeably worse.

If you get any of these, see your doctor as soon as possible.

7

Do You Have Abdominal Pain?

It is pain in the gut that drives most people with an irritable bowel to the doctor. This pain is generally low down on the left-hand side, but it could be in the centre or on the right. It may range from a dull ache to pain of such severity that the sufferer is doubled up, and may even go to a hospital accident and emergency department. It may last from a few minutes to many hours, and may be spasmodic or persistent. Once again, there is such a range of different symptoms that it's not surprising it has taken so many years to piece everything together into one recognized condition.

The pain of IBS is generally colicky, cramp-like, and comes in spasms. The spasm may affect the whole bowel or just one section, so the position and intensity of the pain may vary. People with IBS will typically describe the pain as 'sharp', 'stabbing', 'knife-like', 'burning', 'cutting', 'very strong'. Some find their pain comes on after meals; those with diarrhoea often find the pain comes on with the bowel movement, and then gets better; those with constipation usually find that the pain only gets better when they stop being constipated. When the colon is distended (enlarged and stretched), as happens with constipation, this can produce pain in some unlikely parts of the body – the back, shoulders, thigh and genital area. And, in contrast with this, some people with IBS find they get very little pain, just the other main symptoms.

This chapter suggests ways of coping with abdominal pain. First get it checked by the doctor. It is important to be sure it is IBS and not something else. Once you have your diagnosis, try these various ideas, and see which works best for you:

- Anti-spasmodic drugs, as prescribed by the doctor.
- Homoeopathic nux vomica 6 or 30. Take two tablets one night, two the following morning, and two the following night, then stop. You should notice an improvement in two to four weeks; if your IBS recurs later, repeat this dose. (Homoeopathy is discussed in Chapter 21.)
- When the pain strikes you, breathe deeply, concentrating on the passage of air in your nostrils, and focusing your attention on a point between your eyebrows at the top of your nose; exhale

slowly. Make sure you keep your abdominal muscles relaxed all the time – do not tense them up.

- Lie flat, perhaps with your arms over your head if this feels comfortable, with a hot water bottle on your tummy. You may also find it helpful to use an electric blanket, though you should take great care when doing so.
- Lie on your front with your knees drawn up to your chest, arms straight by your sides, head curled inwards or turned to one side.
- Lie on your back on the floor, head raised on a few books, knees drawn up and feet flat on the floor.
- Use a hot compress – take a small towel, wring it out in hot water, fold to a convenient size, and leave on your abdomen until it cools.
- Be active, go for a walk, do some gentle stretching exercises. If you are in bed, or in a chair, get up and walk around vigorously.
- Get rid of the constipation that might be the cause of the stomach pain (see Chapter 8).
- Do something to take your mind off it. If you have ever attended ante-natal classes, practise the labour-pain exercises you learned. Otherwise, do something, anything, that takes up all your concentration, and makes you think of something else.
- Avoid antacid indigestion tablets. Their high alkaline content destroys the stomach's natural acids that digest food, and if you take these tablets too often the stomach responds by producing extra acid which can cause more pain, more digestive problems, and eventually even a gastric ulcer.
- Infuse 10–20 grams of hops (available from home brewing shops) in 1 litre of boiling water for ten minutes, and drink a cupful after meals.
- Infuse 10–20 grams of balm or lemon balm in the same way, and drink a cupful with meals.
- Heat a teaspoonful of fennel seeds in a cupful of milk, and drink fairly hot.
- In cooking use herbs which aid digestion, and tone and soothe the gut: cumin, fennel, garlic, marjoram, mint, parsley, rosemary, sage, and thyme.
- Infuse 5 grams of lavender in a litre of boiling water; leave for five minutes, strain, and drink three cups a day between meals.
- Infuse 4 or 5 leaves of mint (dried or fresh) in a cup of boiling water, leave for five minutes, strain and drink twice a day after meals. If this causes insomnia, use only two leaves per cup, and

drink one cupful a day, in the morning. You could also use peppermint essence in a glass of warm water.

- Infuse 20–30 grams of fresh or dried thyme in 1 litre of water for about five minutes. Strain, and drink three cupfuls a day after meals.

Most of these ingredients should be available from wholefood or healthfood shops, or large supermarkets.

The following homeopathic remedies may help *cramping pains*:

- Belladonna: if you feel distended, and better when doubled up.
- Bryonia: if you feel better when lying still, and worse from heat.
- Colocynth: if you can't keep still, and feel better when doubled up.
- Magnesia phosphorica: if you feel better for applying heat to your abdomen.

If the pain is caused by *wind*, try the following ideas:

- Take steps to avoid constipation; Chapter 8 has lots of suggestions. A blocked rectum prevents gas escaping that way, so it has no alternative but to build up in the tubes of the abdomen, causing discomfort. By keeping your rectum comparatively empty you allow that gas to escape.
- When the wind builds up, sit up straight, or stand up straight, and if possible walk about vigorously.
- You may find a low-fibre diet helpful: more peeled vegetables, fish, lean meat, white rice, bread and pasta, and less wholemeal bread or pasta, pulses, cereals and dried fruit.
- Be aware that you may be swallowing excess air as you eat or drink and avoid doing this.
- Infuse a cut root of angelica in boiling water for several minutes, strain, and drink a small glassful before meals.
- Chew raw angelica root or leaves.
- Chew mustard seeds with plenty of water.
- Put a few drops of peppermint essence in warm water, and sip.
- Suck sweets containing oil of peppermint.
- Chew charcoal biscuits, or charcoal tablets.
- Add a teaspoon of cinnamon or nutmeg to warm milk; sweeten with honey, and drink.
- Infuse any of the following in boiling water for about 10 minutes,

and drink when it has cooled slightly (you may prefer the drink to be sweetened with honey): marjoram, grated ginger root, fresh or dried basil leaves, half a fresh lemon.

And, finally, some exercises for general improvement of the abdomen:

- This exercise strengthens all the abdominal muscles with the minimum of strain. Lie on your back with knees bent, feet flat on the floor. Clasp your hands behind your head, resting your head on your hands. Gently begin to sit up, without putting strain on your neck, raising yourself about 2–3 inches (5–8 cm) until your shoulder blades are just off the floor. Hold this position for 5 seconds, or longer. Breathe deeply. Repeat several times. Listen to your body, and when your muscles ache it's time to stop.
- Lie on your back with your knees bent and your feet flat on the floor close up to your buttocks. Lift your hips off the floor, drawing the abdominal muscles up and in at the same time. Then lower your hips. Repeat several times, and stop when you feel tired.
- Stand with legs apart, knees bent, hands pressing on thighs. As you breathe in, pull your abdominal muscles in and up, hold your breath, and pump your belly in and out using your muscles. Stop pumping when you need to breathe out, take a normal breath, then breathe in, and repeat. Aim to do 10–15 pumpings at a time.
- Self-help massage of the colon: lie on your back on a flat surface, and roll a tennis ball firmly up the right side of the abdomen, across the bottom of the ribcage, and down the left-hand side (that is, in the direction the digested food travels). This exercise is particularly effective if you do it first thing in the morning before rising.
- Cup one hand with fingers and thumbs closed tightly enough as if you were holding water in your hand, then, keeping the hand in this position 'strike' your colon rhythmically with the hollowed hand and fingertips, keeping the wrists as loose as possible palm facing downwards. As in the previous exercise, work up the right side of the abdomen, across the middle, and down the left side. Do this exercise lying down.

8
Do You Have Constipation?

The symptoms of IBS are much more common in people with long-standing constipation than in most other people. In fact, when people who do not have IBS are deliberately made constipated during research experiments, they start to develop some of the usual symptoms of an irritable bowel; when their constipation is artificially ended by laxatives, their IBS symptoms cease.

Many people with IBS find constipation is their main symptom, either constantly or intermittently. In addition, they will probably have pain in the stomach, because the more constipated a person is, the more likely he or she is to have abdominal pain.

One of the main causes of IBS is an irregularity in the speed with which food passes through the digestive system – too slowly and you get constipation, too quickly and you get diarrhoea.

What is constipation? Most people who get constipation would probably say that the stools are difficult to push out, that even after a bowel movement they have the feeling there is more to come, and that they don't go as often as they think they should. Most doctors would agree it is straining to pass the stools, having less than three bowel movements a week, and passing small, hard stools.

While most people have about one bowel movement a day, some go every 2 or 3 days, some once a week. As a general rule, if you go not more often than twice a day or so, and not less often than about twice a week, that is quite normal, provided that you pass a soft well-formed motion effortlessly without pain or straining.

Generally your bowel habits should remain fairly constant throughout life, changing only when you have a change of environment, such as going on holiday, or eating different food. If your bowel pattern remains unchanged, it is unlikely you have any disease of the digestive system. But if you have more constipation or more diarrhoea and it is not connected with a change in your lifestyle and this change lasts for several weeks, it might be a good idea to see your doctor.

People with IBS often describe their bowel movements as 'like rabbit pellets', or 'small lumpy stools', or 'stringy', or 'hard and dry'. Let us look at why this happens.

In the normal colon, faeces are propelled along by peristalsis, in much the same way as food in propelled down the oesophagus (gullet) towards the stomach (remind yourself of your digestive system by looking at the diagram on page 23). The muscle walls of the colon work best when they are propelling faeces which are soft and bulky; this keeps the muscle walls a regular distance apart (remember, the colon is a tube). Now if the faeces are small and hard, the colon must squeeze in further than its muscular walls can comfortably manage, which causes a build-up of pressure in the colon, and pain as the muscle goes into spasm.

When the muscle is in spasm it no longer propels the faeces in smooth waves towards the rectum. Instead, it just keeps on squeezing and relaxing, often causing quite intense pain. And instead of the faeces moving evenly on their way, they become compressed, and divided into very small segments with each squeeze, causing the typical hard 'pellety' stools of IBS.

Many people remain constipated for years. As a result, they are more likely to get diverticulosis, piles (haemorrhoids), and varicose veins. They may also have lower back pain or stomach ache from a rectum that is always too full with hard compacted faeces, not to mention extra problems like headaches, lethargy, loss of appetite, and a general feeling of being 'under the weather'.

In addition, because food remains so much longer than normal in the digestive system, there is more chance for harmful bacteria to build up and be absorbed into the bloodstream. With most people, food remains in the gut for about one-and-a-half to two-and-a-half days; for those who are constipated, 5 days is average, and it may even be double that. It is not at all unknown for people to go about a month without a bowel movement.

What causes constipation? As with most conditions, there are many causes. The commonest are:

- lack of exercise;
- not enough dietary fibre in the diet;
- ignoring the call to empty the bowel;
- taking certain drugs;
- some medical conditions.

Many drugs cause it, so if you are taking any of these and constipation is a problem to you, talk to your doctor about it:

- painkillers (particularly the strong ones);

- anti-convulsants (used in epilepsy and similar conditions);
- tranquillisers and anti-depressants;
- water-reducing drugs (for heart conditions);
- iron tablets;
- drugs for high blood pressure.

Indigestion tablets can also cause constipation, leading to a vicious circle: you have a pain in your stomach, so you take indigestion tablets, so you may become more constipated, so you get more stomach ache.

Lastly, one of the main causes of constipation is, ironically, over-use of laxatives (see Chapter 10).

If constipation is your problem, here is what you can do about it. The rules are quite simple, and for most people they will do the trick.

- The most natural treatment for simple constipation is a high-fibre diet. Read Chapter 9 for more on this, and also Chapter 12 on the relationship between IBS and food.
- Drink plenty of fluids, preferably non-alcoholic, and sometimes warmed; aim for about 3 pints of fluid a day. Tannin in tea tends to constipate, so drink a herb tea instead; there are some delicious ones available and if you find them a bit sharp, try adding honey.
- It is possible that some foods make your IBS worse. If you suspect this may be so, try the simple diet on p. 47 in order to identify which these foods may be.
- When you eat, a 'food now entering stomach' message is sent to the brain. Then the brain sends a message to the intestines saying 'make room for an incoming meal'. This message causes the large bowel to empty its contents into the storage depot of the rectum to make way for the next meal. So try to empty the bowel just after meals when your body is preparing to move each batch of food on to the next stage. This system works most effectively after the first meal of the day, so be particularly aware of it after breakfast.
- Allow plenty of time for each bowel movement. Try getting up 20 minutes earlier in the morning, eat a leisurely breakfast, then disappear to the toilet with a book, magazine or newspaper for at least 10–15 minutes. Don't push or strain as this could cause piles (haemorrhoids), just allow time for the rectum to become empty.

- An early morning train, bus or car journey may reduce the natural morning urge to empty the bowels. So either fit in time for a long visit to the toilet before your morning journey, or allow time for it when you arrive. A hot drink on the journey may help to get your insides moving.
- Never neglect the urge to 'go'. When the rectum is comfortably full, the stools are covered with slimy mucus to make them easier to pass. But if the stools remain too long in the rectum, this mucus is absorbed back into the body, making the stools hard, dry and painful to pass. So when your body says 'go', then go! That way you work *with* your body, not against it.
- As exercise is one of the things that triggers the bowel to empty, take plenty of it, giving your brain a chance to send 'exercise' messages to the bowel. It needn't be wildly energetic, a brisk walk every day is fine for most people. Exercise also improves your capacity to withstand stress, and keeps your inside muscles in good condition. Many digestive ailments are caused because muscles in the abdomen are too slack, so they sag, and the contents of the abdomen are compressed downwards. This produces congestion, sluggish bowel movements, and constipation.

Here are some traditional remedies for constipation:

- Eat a raw apple in its skin for breakfast every day.
- Infuse $\frac{1}{10}$–$\frac{1}{5}$ ounce (3–5 grams) of basil leaves or flowering tips in boiling water. Strain and drink. Basil also has anti-spasmodic properties.
- Simmer 2 pounds (1 kg) of carrots in 2 pints (1 litre) water for about 1–2 hours. Blend in a liquidizer, or rub through a sieve. Take as a soup.
- Soak figs or prunes overnight in water. The figs can be eaten uncooked, but prunes should be cooked before eating. Drink the water they have been cooked in, too.
- Eat kiwi fruit, a traditional remedy from New Zealand, from time to time.
- Eat charcoal biscuits (obtainable from chemists or health-food shops).
- Take natural liquorice, as sweets or in stick form.
- Massage your lower back with a blend of essential oils: 20 drops of marjoram plus 5 drops of rose in 2 fluid ounces (50 ml) of vegetable oil. Essential oils can be obtained from many healthfood shops.

9
The Role of Fibre

This chapter will interest mainly those who have as their main IBS symptom constipation, or stomach pain due to constipation, or constipation which alternates with diarrhoea.

You will remember that the large intestine, or colon, is a tube with muscular walls. The muscles of this tube work best if they are able to propel soft bulky stools in a wave-like movement (peristalsis) down to the storage depot of the rectum. The muscles move to compress the bowel contents, but if these are already compressed hard and dry the natural activity of the bowel is largely wasted. Pressure builds up in the colon, causing pain and discomfort anywhere in the abdomen. Therefore, it's important to do everything you can to keep the contents of the bowel soft and bulky, and the simplest and most effective way to do this is to eat plenty of 'dietary fibre' or 'roughage'.

Dietary fibre is the material that makes up the cell walls of plants; it contains substances called cellulose, lignin and polysaccharides. It is found in the skin, husks and leaves of plants. If you were a rabbit or a cow or a caterpillar you would eat large quantities of green material such as grass and leaves, and you would have in your gut the necessary enzymes to break it down in your digestive system, and it would do you a power of good.

But we human beings don't have these enzymes in our bodies, and so can't digest dietary fibre. It just passes straight through us unchanged and undigested. Until quite recently, the received wisdom was that if it passed straight through then it couldn't be doing any good, so there wasn't much point in eating it. Now we know better.

Because dietary fibre is not digested and absorbed, it ends up in the large intestine much as it entered the mouth. It is bulky so it makes stools bulkier, so the stools fill out the tubular bowel, so the bowel muscles have something to work on, so pressure doesn't build up causing pain and spasm. Dietary fibre also softens the stools, making them easy to pass. In addition, it allows the stools to hold more water in the bowel, so they become less dry.

All in all, dietary fibre is a remarkable substance, and if you have simple constipation which is not caused by serious disease, a

39

high-fibre diet will relieve it and prevent it recurring. If, as part of a 'civilised' Western diet, you eat white bread, processed foods, bland foods, and not much fresh fruit and vegetables, don't be surprised if you get constipation. You are eating very little dietary fibre.

Rural Africans eat large quantities of fruit and vegetables which are full of fibre. Researchers have found that the average rural African produces a large quantity of soft stools, that food passes through the gut in about 36 hours or less, and that constipation, IBS, diverticular disease and similar problems are almost unknown.

The average Westerner, by contrast, produces small quantities of fairly hard stools, and our food takes several days to pass through the gut. Hence the digestive disorders common in Western society.

So, from now on, eat:

- wholemeal, wheatmeal or granary bread instead of white;
- high-fibre breakfast cereals, muesli, and those containing bran;
- plenty of fruit and vegetables, eating the skins wherever possible –as cooking can break down the fibre of fruit and vegetables, eat these either raw or only lightly cooked;
- plenty of dried fruit (raisins, prunes, apricots, figs, etc.);
- baked beans, processed peas;
- home-made soups instead of tinned or packet;
- wholemeal pasta (spaghetti, macaroni), and pulses (like lentils, peas and beans – kidney, soya, haricot, butter, broad, mung, etc.).

In addition, have you tried bran? Even Hippocrates (often called the father of medicine) in the fourth century BC, was aware that bran bulked stools. Then we forgot all about it for two thousand years or so, and now it is back in fashion. It really can work wonders for constipation – though it would not appear in any list of 'My Favourite Foods'.

The easiest way to take bran is to start with one dessertspoon (12 ml) of raw bran a day – perhaps on a high-fibre breakfast cereal or in soup or stewed fruit, or mixed with fruit juice. Raw unprocessed bran is more effective than cooked bran, but if you find it really difficult to take, bran in the form of high-fibre breakfast cereals is next best. Also, coarse flaky bran is more effective than fine powdery bran, but less palatable.

Most bran is derived from wheat, and if you have an intolerance to wheat it may disagree with you. If so, see if you can get rice bran or soya bran from your chemist or wholefood shop. Even if you are not affected by wheat you may find these other forms of bran more effective.

Gradually increase the amount of bran you take, until you can pass a soft stool without effort. If your bowels become upset, reduce the dose slightly, but don't stop. You may get some wind and bloating, but eventually you should be able to find the daily level of bran that gives you a comfortable bowel movement without wind.

Too much bran can cause you to feel bloated, full of wind, and generally uncomfortable, so don't overdo it or you may feel worse. If you are taking bran, drinking at least 3 pints of water a day may help. It is also suggested that, if you have a lot of wind, eating orange peel helps the smell!

(A note here about fibre and wind. As with so many things, there seem to be two schools of thought. One says that wind is made worse by constipation, so eat a high-fibre diet to get rid of the constipation and the wind should be much improved. The other says that a high-fibre diet makes wind worse, so have a low-fibre diet. So if you have excessive wind, why not try each method for about a month and see which works best for you?)

Bran is not the easiest stuff to take, some people just can't seem to eat it, and for some it doesn't work at all. So if you are one of these, make sure you eat plenty of all those other high-fibre foods, especially fruit and vegetables. If you can eat raw vegetables, so much the better; this doesn't mean just celery, carrots and salads, but also raw cauliflower, mushrooms, sprouts, broccoli, green beans and courgettes.

Your doctor may be able to prescribe a bulking agent such as Isogel or Fybogel. This has the same effect of bulking out the stools, making them soft and easy to pass, and may reduce stomach pain. But if you can help yourself with diet, this is surely better than relying long-term on a doctor's prescriptions.

Finally, fibre has other advantages unrelated to IBS: it fills you up more than highly refined foods do, so you eat less, so you may keep your weight down; it can help prevent diseases such as gallstones, diverticular disease, diabetes which starts in adulthood, coronary heart disease, and bloodclots following surgery. A high-fibre diet also reduces the risk of bowel and colon cancer, both of which are associated with the high-fat, low-fibre diet so common in our Western civilization; this is possibly because, by speeding up the passage of waste materials through the gut, potentially harmful cancer-forming substances do not hang around long enough to do damage.

Dietary fibre affects nearly every function of the large intestine: it increases the bulk of the faeces, reduces the length of time waste materials stay in the gut, softens faeces, eases bowel movements, and reduces pressure. So as pressure causes pain, and fibre reduces pressure, it's got to be a Good Thing.

10

Beware of Laxatives

Many people use larger and larger quantities of ever-stronger laxatives more and more often, to less and less effect. They are afraid to stop in case they get more constipated. Yet one of the main reasons for constipation is over-use of laxatives.

Laxatives are among the commonest medicines bought over the counter; in addition to this, millions of laxatives are prescribed by doctors. Possibly up to 30% of the general population use them regularly. This is not only expensive, it is unnecessary and potentially harmful. And you would be surprised how many people with IBS regularly take laxatives and prefer not to tell their doctor.

Laxatives are extensively misused in the mistaken belief that there is some wondrous relationship between good health and a daily emptying of the bowels – 'regularity is next to godliness'. This just isn't so. As you will have read in Chapter 8, it is quite normal to have a bowel movement 2 or 3 times a day or 2 or 3 times a week. Even going one or two days over what is normal for you is nothing to worry about. As long as your movement is soft, well formed, easy to pass, and the same as it has always been, that's how it should be, and you are quite normal.

There really is no known connection between a daily bowel movement and good health. Nor does a less regular pattern mean poor health, unless it is recent, persists for several weeks, or has a noticeable effect on your life.

Reading advertisements for laxatives and health salts (whose manufacturers are, after all, trying to sell as much of their product as possible), it is easy to get the impression that missing a bowel movement is something really serious. So you become worried, and take a laxative. This empties the whole of the large intestine, and several days pass before a normal quantity of stool forms again. In the meantime you don't have another bowel movement because there's nothing in the bowel to pass, so you think you are constipated, and you take laxatives again. Thus you never give your body a chance to work normally. If this pattern continues, eventually the bowel muscle becomes damaged, and won't work at all unless there is a laxative to force it into action.

Ideally the rectum will empty almost completely every day or so, as will about one-third of the contents of the large intestine. To empty everything all at once is not what the system was designed to do.

If you do take laxatives or health salts regularly, don't rush to cut down on them. Reduce the dose gradually, perhaps from two doses a day to one dose a day for a few days, then one dose every other day for several days, then two doses a week, then one dose a week, until you can finally stop completely without a shock to your system.

There are several kinds of laxative on the market. Some add bulk to the faeces to make the bowel muscle propel them more easily; others loosen and lubricate the faeces; others stimulate and irritate the bowel. The main types are:

- *Bulk-forming laxatives*, usually made from fibre such as ispaghula husks (brand names are Fybogel, Isogel, Metamucil, Normacol and Regulan). These are the ones most commonly prescribed for IBS, and the safest for long-term use. They stimulate the bowel muscles naturally by making the stools moist, soft, bulky and easier to pass. Take plenty of fluids with them, as fluid keeps the laxative soft and prevents it from becoming sticky. (They may also help prevent diverticulitis.)
- *Lubricant laxatives* such as liquid paraffin. If you take these regularly your body may fail to absorb some essential vitamins; they can also cause trouble with the gut wall, liver and spleen. Liquid paraffin coats some of the food, preventing its being properly digested and absorbed; it also prevents useful bacteria from working, it does not mix with water so does not soften the faeces, and if you use it regularly it may leak out through the rectum.
- *Stimulant laxatives* such as cascara, castor oil and senna. They increase bowel movements by irritating the lining of the bowel, and stimulating the bowel muscles to contract. However, from reading the chapter on constipation, you will know that it can be very painful if the walls of the bowel contract further than they comfortably can onto hard compacted stools. If you have IBS, it is likely that your colon (or bowel) already contracts at a higher than normal rate, so laxatives of this type will probably make your stomach pain worse. Stimulant laxatives can also be dangerous if, for any reason, you have an obstructed bowel.
- *Saline laxatives*, often called 'health salts', make the stools bulkier by causing them to retain water (unlike bulk-forming

44

laxatives which make stools bulkier by causing them to retain dietary fibre). To do this they may draw fluids from the body, causing it to become dehydrated. They may be harmful to people with kidney disease, or on diuretics (water-reducing drugs commonly prescribed for heart conditions); if in doubt, ask your doctor whether health salts are a good idea for you. He may suggest you take Lactulose instead, which works in a similar way and is preferable.

Finally, don't take laxatives to relieve pain in the stomach, or cramp, or colic. These pains may signal a more serious condition like acute appendicitis.

11
Do You Have Diarrhoea?

As you will know by now, diarrhoea is one of the main symptoms of IBS. You may have it on its own, or alternating with constipation, and with or without mucus. The usual pattern is to have a period of constipation with the typical 'rabbit pellets', then out it all comes as a rather 'explosive' diarrhoea.

In fact this is not typical diarrhoea. Typical (or *infective*) diarrhoea – also known as gastro-enteritis, Spanish tummy, Delhi belly, etc. – is usually caused by an infection, or by taking contaminated food or water, and produces the typical 'upset stomach' – vomiting, abdominal pain, and great quantities of very loose stools as the body tries to get rid of whatever has contaminated it. You will probably feel dreadful, all limp and washed out, but when you have got rid of it all, you will start to feel better again.

The diarrhoea of IBS is rather different. The quantity of faeces that you pass is much less than with infective diarrhoea; in fact over several days it is much the same quantity as any other person's motions, though more frequent and sloppy. And it is not caused by any infection or contamination.

With the diarrhoea form of IBS, you will probably get it worse in the morning, and feel more settled as the day progresses. The pain may get worse as you have a bowel movement, and then disappear. Also, you may have to get up in the night with it. Some people have IBS and diarrhoea without any pain at all. Once again, there are so many variations that it's not surprising it has taken so long to link all the symptoms together.

It is possible that part of your colon does not work as well as it should, and passes food on to the rectum before all the water has been properly absorbed, making the stools fairly runny instead of fairly dry. Also, your own rectum may not like being even half-full, and may send 'emptying' messages rather too early.

Also bear in mind that quite a large number of those with the diarrhoea form of IBS use laxatives regularly and surreptitiously, and this is probably one of the causes of the problem.

Researchers have discovered that 50–60% of individuals with the diarrhoea form of IBS have an intolerance to one or more foods. You may be one of these if you:

- have diarrhoea as your main symptom;
- wake at night needing to have a bowel movement;
- started to get IBS after an attack of gastro-enteritis or a long course of antibiotics;
- feel very tired and weary;
- get headaches.

Whether diet is or is not an important cause of your IBS, those who have the diarrhoea form of the condition generally have more anxiety than those with the constipation form. After all, from those butterflies in the tummy before an important event, you will be aware of the link between diarrhoea and anxiety. So take positive steps to reduce stress and anxiety as a good way to helping your irritable bowel. Later chapters on stress contain lots of ideas.

Here are some other well-tried remedies for diarrhoea:

- Strange as it may seem, the same high-fibre/low-fat diet which is recommended for constipation, also works for diarrhoea in many people. Bran may work for you, although it may make the stools sticky for a few weeks.
- Bulk laxatives (such as Fybogel or Isogel) help bind loose stools together.
- Anti-diarrhoea drugs prescribed by the doctor can be of great benefit, particularly if you get so agitated about being far from the toilet that your whole life is seriously restricted.
- Mix 1 dessertspoon (12 ml) of cider vinegar in a glass of water and drink before each meal.
- Mix one heaped dessertspoon (15 ml) of arrowroot (obtainable from chemists) with a small quantity of cold water until smooth. Top up with about 1 pint of boiling water, and drink when cool. You may prefer it flavoured, with blackcurrant juice for example.

12

You Are What You Eat

Do onions make your irritable bowel worse? Or oranges, or cabbage, or coffee? Or perhaps milk, beer, breakfast cereals or fried food? If so, take comfort – you are just like lots of other people who have IBS. A recent report by the Royal College of Physicians accepts that food can be the cause of several conditions, including IBS. Perhaps 20% of people with this condition have some form of food intolerance, especially if their IBS is characterized by diarrhoea. It really *isn't* 'all in the mind'.

Nowadays the typical British diet might include white bread, cornflakes, cakes, biscuits, chocolate, pies, chips, frozen vegetables, tinned fruit, tea, coffee, squash, and immense quantities of processed foods. Two hundred years ago most of these were quite unknown to the general population, and so was IBS. Could there be a connection?

We eat about twice the quantity of carbohydrates (including sugar) that we need in our less active lives, and half the fibre. We probably eat a lot more fat than is good for us, and an amazing cocktail of chemicals in processed food. Is it surprising that things start to go wrong inside our insides? In addition, most of us have been prescribed antibiotics at some time or other, sometimes quite frequently or for extended periods, and this may affect the balance of bacteria in the gut, killing off some useful bacteria and altering others so that they cause chemicals to be produced that aggravate IBS.

Although some GPs and gastro-enterologists still firmly believe IBS is due almost entirely to psychological factors, this is not really fair. However, some of their patients are convinced their IBS occurs because they are 'allergic' to certain foods, when in fact what they have is an *intolerance* to these foods. Let us look at the difference between these two.

With an *allergy*, you develop abnormal antibodies to substances (such as pollen or the house dust mite), called 'allergens'. The antibodies react against these allergens, producing allergic symptoms such as wheezing and a runny nose. When you develop antibodies against a particular food, the food becomes the allergen and the antibodies combine with that food to trigger off cells which produce chemicals such as histamines, again producing typical allergic symptoms. (Doctors often prescribe anti-histamines to overcome these unpleasant symptoms) This is a true food allergy, and can be clearly detected by well-established medical testing.

Intolerance is a much wider term. The food may cause unpleasant symptoms, but all medical allergy tests prove negative, so the doctor may think his patient is imagining it all. Yet some foods contain chemicals which upset some people. We all have beneficial bacteria which are busy working in the digestive system, and antibiotics can kill some of these off. They are then replaced by other bacteria which react differently in the gut and produce chemicals which cause unpleasant symptoms to develop. Damage to the intestines by infection or inflammation can also cause food intolerance; suddenly you are sensitive to foods that never bothered you before.

Foods which typically aggravate the symptoms of an irritable bowel are: wheat, corn, dairy products, coffee, oats, rye, tea, citrus fruits, fatty and fried foods, onions, cabbage, salads, and alcohol. Smoking can also have this effect.

Wheat is one of the commonest foods to aggravate IBS, and people who have an intolerance to wheat often also can't take corn. Unfortunately wheat is in so many products that it is not easy to cut it down. Many health-food and wholefood shops sell products that do not contain wheat. These products are manufactured mainly for people with coeliac disease (who are unable to absorb the gluten in wheat), but you could try them and see if they are an acceptable wheat substitute for you.

Dairy products are the next most common problem foods. They include not only milk, butter, cheese and yoghurt, but also many processed and packet foods. Look at the list of ingredients on packets of biscuits, margarine, cereals, puddings, sauces, sweets, and you will probably see whey, whey solids, milk solids, and skimmed milk powder, which all come from milk.

Milk contains a sugar called lactose, which is broken down in the gut by an enzyme called lactase. Some people (especially those with the diarrhoea form of IBS) don't produce enough lactase, so can't properly break down the lactose in milk products. Because of this, they get diarrhoea.

Where irritable bowel is characterized by pain after meals, you may find it helpful to eat less fat and more protein, as fats can cause the muscles of the intestines to go into painful spasm.

Some people feel they are so sensitive to so many foods that their lives become nothing but misery. They never eat out at friends' homes, or in restaurants; they avoid functions that include meals; they may even stop going on holiday; and they eat intolerably restricted diets. Their own lives, and their families' lives, become dominated by their irritable bowels.

A report on food additives presented to the Royal College of Physicians in 1988 produced some interesting results, suggesting that people may not be sensitive to nearly as many foods as they fear. During experiments, when people knew they were eating something that typically disagreed with them, they got unpleasant reactions. When they ate the same substances without knowing what they were eating, very few got unpleasant reactions. This, so far, is what other researchers have discovered. But the researchers in this experiment carried the tests further, and came to the conclusion that if you eat something you know will disagree with you, a certain level of anxiety is generated which causes changes to take place in your body; these changes disrupt the digestive process, and cause the unpleasant reactions.

This does *not* mean that you are neurotic, or obsessive, or over anxious. There is, indeed, a direct physical change taking place; it is not imaginary. But it is yet another example of how your state of mind is contributing directly to your irritable bowel. Now that you know about it, you are in a position to do all you can to prevent it.

Many people find that if they eat a lot of one food it affects them badly, as if there is a limit to the quantity of that particular food that their body can tolerate. If they can keep below the threshold that causes problems, they are often all right. Sometimes the answer is to cut it out altogether for a while, give your body time to get used to being without it, then to eat it only occasionally, or in small quantities. Once you can accept that you can eat it in small quantities without an unpleasant reaction, your level of anxiety about that food will fall, and you may then be able to eat more than you realized.

In order to discover which foods disagree with you, as a first step try this simple regime. For two weeks cut out completely all red meat, fatty foods, fried foods, coffee, and alcohol, and no more than about two other things that you know for certain make your irritable bowel worse. In addition, have as little dairy produce as you can. Just cutting out these things may make your IBS better enough to live with. Have a simple leisurely breakfast of fruit juice, cereal, and wholemeal toast with vegetable margarine and marmalade or honey. For lunch (or supper) have wholemeal bread sandwiches, or salad, and fresh fruit. For supper (or lunch) have a vegetarian meal, or fish, chicken or lean meat with salad or fresh vegetables, followed by fresh fruit. Drink as little tea and coffee as you can, and try to cut out alcohol and smoking; use honey instead of sugar for sweetening. If this makes you feel better, try introducing other foods in small quantities at the rate of one every two days, noting any reactions these new foods provoke. With any luck this slightly reduced diet should show up which foods are causing problems, and you can adapt your eating habits accordingly.

However if after two weeks on this diet you still have all the symptoms as badly as ever and you are in good health, put aside about a month of your life to try the following method. If you can persevere, you will have taken positive steps to improve your irritable bowel . Don't try this if you are pregnant or frail, or have diabetes, anorexia nervosa, kidney disease, or any other serious health problem. If in doubt, ask your doctor. In addition, work on reducing the level of stress in your life; this is one of the most effective ways to reduce IBS.

On Day One, eat what you would normally eat, and have a large (but not over-large) supper.

On Day Two, go on a total fast. Fasting is a good way to clear toxins from the body. Drink as much water as you need, but don't eat anything unless you start to feel decidedly unwell; in that case have some cooked white fish (*not* fried) and perhaps a banana. Do not drive, or do anything physically demanding. You may get a headache, but don't take anything for it, as it is a sign that the body is getting rid of the toxins; just leave nature to work in your best interests. You will probably find it easier to fast on a day when you are not at work or doing anything energetic.

On Day Three, start the following short-term exclusion diet. It has been developed by Addenbrooke's Hospital in Cambridge for those with food intolerances. It is a healthy diet, it includes plenty of fresh and wholesome foods, and it works well with IBS. I am grateful to Dr John Hunter of Addenbrooke's Hospital for permission to use details of the diet he and his colleagues find so helpful for their patients.

For two weeks eat only the foods listed in the 'Allowed' column of Table 1, and none of the foods in the 'Not allowed' column. You should be aware that many of these substances appear in lots of

Table 1. Foods for the Addenbrooke's exclusion diet

	Not allowed	Allowed
Meat	preserved meats, bacon, sausages	all other meats
Fish	smoked fish, shell fish	white fish
Vegetables	potatoes, onions, sweetcorn	all other vegetables, salads, pulses, swede and parsnip
Fruit	citrus fruit, e.g., oranges, grapefruit	all other fruit, e.g., apples, bananas, pears
Cereals	wheat, oats, barley, rye, corn	rice, ground rice, rice flakes, rice flour, sago, Rice Krispies, tapioca, millet, buckwheat, rice cakes
Cooking oils	corn oil, vegetable oil	sunflower oil, soya oil, safflower oil, olive oil
Dairy products	cow's milk, butter, most margarines, cow's milk yoghurt and cheese, eggs	goat's milk, soya milk, sheep's milk, Tomor margarine, goat's and sheep's milk yoghurt and cheese, soya cheese
Beverages	tea, coffee (beans, instant and decaffeinated), fruit squashes, orange juice, grapefruit juice, alcohol, tap water	herbal teas, e.g., camomile, fresh fruit juices, e.g., apple, pineapple, tomato juice, mineral, distilled or deionized water
Miscellaneous	chocolates, yeast, preservatives	carob, sea salt, herbs, spices; in moderation: sugar, honey

everyday foods. For example, wheat is an ingredient of bread, batter, meat pies, packet soups, sausages, stock cubes, crispbreads, and so on. Yeast is an ingredient of bread (except soda bread), yoghurt, wine, beer, overripe fruit, vinegar, and vitamin B products. So check food labels most carefully. (Fuller details of foods and additives to be wary of on a restricted diet, together with lots of suitable recipes, are given in *The Allergy Diet*, and its successor *The Food Intolerance Diet Book*, both by Elizabeth Workman, Dr Virginia Alun Jones and Dr John Hunter, both published by Dunitz.)

Keep strictly to this diet for two weeks. If you take a day off, start again from the beginning. At the end of this chapter are some sample meals to get you started. During this time keep a record of everything you eat, together with any symptoms you have, and when. If you get an unpleasant symptom it will probably have been caused by something you ate in the previous 24 hours.

After two weeks, you can start to introduce new foods at the rate of one every two days. Again, record all your symptoms. If any new food causes an unpleasant reaction stop taking it, go back to the exclusion diet until the reaction stops, and then introduce foods at the rate of one every two days. Drink plenty of water, but don't take any pills or medicines unless prescribed by your doctor.

Addenbrooke's Hospital recommends you reintroduce foods in the following order: tap water, potatoes, cow's milk, yeast, tea, rye, butter, onions, eggs, oats, coffee, chocolate, barley, citrus fruits, corn, cow's cheese, white wine, shell fish, cow's yoghurt, vinegar, wheat, nuts, preservatives, processed foods.

Bear in mind that it may well be your anxiety about a food that is causing it to disagree with you. If any item sets you back, stop taking it, wait a few days and then try something else. Take things slowly, don't rush. It is possible you may not be able to eat some foods for a long time, so just accept that. Food intolerances can come and go. So if something disagrees with you now, try it again in six months' time, and you may find you can then eat it without problems.

Once you know what you can comfortably eat, try to establish a diet that agrees with you, and that you can live with for as long as necessary – if you set yourself a diet that is too restricted you may fail to keep to it, which will make you feel discouraged, and will probably cause your symptoms to return, or if you do stick at it you may make everyone else's life a misery.

You should notice a definite improvement during the second

week of the diet. If two weeks on the diet brings no improvement, it is likely that your IBS is not caused or triggered by problem foods. So resume normal eating, ask your doctor if he has any other treatment to recommend, or consider some form of alternative therapy (see Chapter 20).

Remember that, for most people, IBS is also related to stress, so learn to relax, and at the same time follow some of the ideas in Chapter 19. There isn't much point in cutting out certain foods if you do not at the same time try to reduce the other main cause of IBS – stress.

Finally, a few tips on how to eat:

- Always eat breakfast, and in a quiet leisurely way. Sit down at a table – no more perching at the breakfast bar. Start the new day feeling relaxed.
- Eat at regular times, and never hurry. Eat slowly, and chew your food thoroughly.
- Leave the table able to eat more. Don't overeat.

A good diet may cost more than a bad one, but poor health is a misery, and totally reduces your joy in life. Consider what you spend on such passing things as your house, your clothes, your car, your hobbies and holidays. Your body has to travel with you till the end of your life, so treat it well, nurture and care for it; it will be time and money well spent.

Sample menus for the Exclusion Diet

Whether you use these menu ideas or not, it is important that for two weeks you keep strictly to the list of foods on page 52. Individual recipes are given for dishes marked with an asterisk in order to avoid the use of dairy or wheat products. If you are out at work at lunchtime, invest in some plastic food storage boxes and select from the list dishes that you could take with you. It's only for about two weeks, so stick to the diet and don't be tempted to eat unsuitable snacks in the middle of the day.

For breakfast (every day) say goodbye to orange juice, corn flakes, bacon and eggs, white toast with butter and marmalade, and coffee. Instead start the day with:

- home-made muesli*;

- stewed fruit (apricots, prunes, apples) with or without goat's milk yoghurt, and sweetened with honey;
- rice crackers, with non-dairy spread and jam or honey;
- Rice Krispies (or any cereal that does not contain wheat, corn, oats or rye – check packet labels carefully), with a milk substitute or fruit juice;
- apple, pineapple or tomato juice;
- herb tea.

For lunch and dinner you might like to try the following:

Day 1 lunch cauliflower in cheese sauce*; raw apple
supper avocado salad, with apple and beetroot in yoghurt dressing*; banana jelly*

Day 2 lunch buckwheat croquettes* with creamed spinach*; melon
supper noodles tossed in non-dairy 'butter', mixed with mushrooms; baked pears with honey

Day 3 lunch home-made soup*; bananas
supper grilled lamb's liver, mushrooms, carrots, cauliflower; baked apple stuffed with sultanas and honey

Day 4 lunch trout or mackerel salad; mixed dried fruit soaked overnight in apple juice
supper leeks/cauliflower/celery/courgettes/green beans (according to season) in cheese sauce*; fresh fruit (not citrus)

Day 5 lunch lentil rissoles (taste better if made the day before); fresh fruit (not citrus)
supper grilled lamb chops and vegetables (not potatoes, onions, cabbage or sweetcorn); rice pudding*

Day 6 lunch chicken with salad of apple, courgette, cauliflower or cucumber; stewed fruit
supper stir fry of sprouting vegetables with any other vegetables except potatoes, cabbage, onions or sweetcorn, and flavoured with tamari; baked bananas (cooked with honey, non-dairy margarine and lemon juice)

Day 7 lunch grilled white fish with vegetables; raw fruit (not citrus)
supper risotto with spinach, left-over chicken, and other vegetables; fresh fruit salad (not citrus)

Recipes

Health-food and wholefood shops, and many large supermarkets, sell a range of soya milks (sweetened, non-sweetened, or flavoured), non-dairy margarines and cheese, goat's milk, cheese and yogurt.

Muesli

Mix together buckwheat (no relation to wheat, despite its name) or millet with dried fruit such as apricots, prunes, raisins, sultanas and chopped apple. Serve with a milk substitute (such as soya milk) and honey.

Cheese sauce

Melt 1 oz (30 g) non-dairy margarine, blend in 1 oz soya flour, cook for about 1 minute, then slowly mix in 10 fl. oz. (300 ml) soya milk, stirring all the time with a wooden spoon. When thoroughly blended add 2–3 oz (60–90 g) non-dairy cheese, and stir until melted.

Yoghurt dressing

Goat's milk yoghurt mixed with chopped mint, chives, garlic and seasoning.

Banana jelly

Sprinkle a sachet of gelatine on 3 fl. oz. (80 ml) of heated apple juice and stir until dissolved. Make up to 1 pint (600 ml) with more apple juice. Add sliced bananas. Leave to set.

Buckwheat croquettes

Cook 6 oz (175 g) buckwheat in twice its own volume of water until the water has been absorbed and the buckwheat is soft; drain and cool. Add finely chopped celery/carrots/leeks, 1 oz. (30 g) soya flour, seasoning and herbs. Shape into rounds ½ inch (1 cm) thick, and fry on both sides until cooked.

Creamed spinach

Cook spinach in a very small quantity of water without salt until it can be easily chopped into a pulp. Add plenty of non-dairy margarine, and seasoning, and mix together until creamy.

Soup

Cook together plenty of suitable vegetables, previously chopped or shredded, with a cup of red lentils, until soft. Mix them all in a blender until the liquid has a soup-like consistency.

Rice pudding

Sprinkle 3 oz (80 g) flaked rice on to 1 pint (600 ml) of near-boiling non-dairy milk. Simmer for 10–15 minutes (or according to directions on packet). Sweeten with honey, and serve alone or with stewed fruit.

Salad dressing

Mix equal parts apple juice and sunflower oil (or according to taste), add parsley/mint/chives as desired.

13
What is Stress?

Does your bowel become more irritable when you are under stress? If so, take comfort: you are not alone.

You may have noticed that whereas one person under stress will develop migraine, another has asthma, someone else gets catarrh, and others suffer from coronary heart disease, ulcers, skin disorders, or irritable bowel syndrome. It would appear that each of us has a 'weak link' – overload it, and it will snap. Most adults, and many children, find there is one particular part of them that always seems to give trouble when they are tired, anxious, run down or under stress of any sort. If you get IBS, then your weak point is probably your gut.

What is stressful for one is perfectly comfortable for another. Everyone is different. But because stress plays such an important part in most people's IBS, three chapters in this book are devoted to it. This chapter explains what stress is, and the next two cover stress as it relates particularly to IBS, and then what you can do about it.

So, what is this intangible thing that upsets your insides, that you can't touch or see, or even describe clearly? The more you know about it, the more you will be able to recognize it and then do something about it.

Long ago, our ancestors lived simple lives in caves. They were without the pressures of the telephone, commuting, traffic hold-ups, demanding jobs, and trying to cope with looking after children while going out to work. The only hold ups they met would be with the greater four-toed mammoth, or something similar.

Now just imagine early Homo Sapiens meeting this mammoth. He may think (in grunts, of course), something like 'This will keep me and the missus in meat and fur for many a moon. I will chase after it. Of course, it may decide I can keep it in meat for a day or so, in which case it will chase after me.' And his body will recognize that either of these events will be decidely stressful, and will prepare itself accordingly.

His brain sends messages to his adrenal glands to produce lots of adrenalin. This causes vital changes to take place to give him a better chance of survival. The blood will drain from his skin and digestive organs, to give more resources to his muscles. Sugars and fats will be

released into his blood to provide much needed energy for all that running. He will breathe faster so more oxygen is made available to burn up the sugar and fat and make it useful quickly. His pupils will enlarge to give him better vision. His blood will thicken so it will coagulate quickly if he is wounded. And his blood pressure will rise as his heart pumps away like crazy keeping the whole body working in overdrive. He is, obviously, very well prepared for fight with the mammoth, or flight away from it.

We have changed a lot in the last few million years. We have moved out of caves, invented computers, landed on the moon, and created designer-label jeans. All very modern. Unfortunately our bodies haven't really kept pace, and in evolutionary terms we are still living in caves.

Like Mr Homo Sapiens, when we are under stress (whether in a traffic jam, or having an argument, or working extra hard, or feeling dreadfully bored, or facing an unhappy marriage or a job we don't like), we get the same changes that prepared him for fight or flight. Extra adrenalin is produced, as a result of which our blood thickens, fats and sugars are released, the digestive system closes down, the heart starts pumping wildly, blood pressure rises, and then . . . nothing. We are still just where we were five minutes ago. No rushing around, no fighting, no action to use up all that adrenalin.

And what happens to all the changes? The blood remains thicker for some time, fats and sugars hang around in the bloodstream, the heart takes time to slow down, and return to its normal pressure. This is the perfect scenario for coronary heart disease and other stress-related illnesses.

There is another effect, too. As well as producing adrenalin, the adrenal glands help the body fight infection. But constant stress produces changes in these glands which reduces their ability to do this. That is why, after periods of stress, many people get colds, feel run down, tired, have aches and pains . . . and digestive disorders. It's all to do with those overloaded adrenal glands. There is also a recognized link between stress and certain types of cancer.

Lots of things cause stress:

- *Obvious things* like marriage problems, job problems, family and personal relationships, changing job, moving house, the death or illness of a close family member, legal procedures, being in debt.
- *Less obvious things* like going on holiday, getting married, becoming a parent, retirement, leaving school, Christmas.

- *Biological changes* such as illness, infection, and taking a long course of drugs.
- *Environmental factors* like noise, poor lighting, pollution, bad equipment design, too much heat or cold.

So it's hardly surprising that there's a lot of it about. And people react quite differently, too. Physical signs of being under stress might be:

- sitting on the edge of a chair;
- disturbed sleep;
- eating, drinking or smoking more;
- talking rapidly;
- nervous twitches;
- tiredness;
- weeping;
- breathlessness;
- chest pains;
- headaches;
- sexual difficulties;
- suffering more illness.

Emotional signs of being under stress are:

- changes in mood;
- feeling unable to cope;
- over-reacting to minor difficulties;
- difficulty in thinking rationally;
- aggression;
- impatience;
- a feeling of failure;
- dreading the future;
- depression or irritability;
- rushing from one job to the next.

Some individuals are more prone to stress than others: especially those who feel they do not have control over their own lives, those with low self-esteem, those who take no exercise, are uncomfortable with change, who eat a poor diet, are overweight, or who smoke. So there's a lot here that you can do to help yourself. Stress itself does not kill – it's how you react to it that is important.

Some people react badly to the stress of overwork, or of boredom, others to the stress of arguments, others to the stress of a change of diet, or to various drugs.

How each person reacts depends on such things as previous experiences, whether this is the first time this particular type of stress has occurred, personality, culture, and basic genetic susceptibility to stress. In fact the damage done to your body depends less on the level of stress, and much more on your ability to cope with it. Some people cope well, take it all in their stride, and genuinely do not seem too bothered by levels of stress which would reduce someone else to a quivering wreck.

This is where the remaining chapters come in useful. You, too, can be the one that copes without problems, once you know what to do.

Taking drugs for stress (except as a very short-term measure) can do more harm than good. For a start, many tranquillisers and antidepressants (as well as alcohol) are addictive, and after a while you may find it extremely hard to give them up. Also, they just mask the unpleasant symptoms without treating the underlying cause, so your stress continues, you lose all motivation to do something about it, and you have to keep taking more and more drugs to achieve the same effect.

In the end, you *must* tackle the *underlying cause*.

14

Stress and Your Irritable Bowel

'The most promising techniques are stress management procedures' (from letter on irritable bowel syndrome in *The Lancet*, 28 September 1985).

Can you remember the first time you were called, in disgrace, to see the headteacher? Or waited for your first job interview? Or played in your first match? Or took part in a play? No doubt lots of feelings jostled for position inside you, and almost certainly one of them was 'butterflies in the tummy'. You may even have had diarrhoea, or complete loss of appetite. All of us notice a connection between fear, emotion, anxiety and how our insides behave, because there are direct links between the brain and the intestines. In addition, if you have IBS, you almost certainly have a bowel that over-reacts to *any* stimulus, whether to certain foods, or to being overloaded as in constipation, or to emotion.

Most people can trace the onset of their irritable bowel to some stressful event such as exams, marital problems, the breakup of a close relationship, financial difficulties or problems at work. Even young adults with IBS generally get it because they find life stressful.

Tests have proved that a distressed mind leads to an over-active colon (bowel). It has not yet been discovered whether IBS patients react differently from other people, or whether they have an unusually direct link between emotion and how the colon works, or whether the colon has become extra-sensitive. But for some reason not yet fully understood, if you have IBS, you are more likely than other people to get digestive problems when you are anxious. It could be caused by the adrenalin that anxiety produces, but no one yet knows for sure.

The digestive systems of those without IBS become less disturbed the longer stress continues; so it could be that the IBS sufferer just fails to adapt in this way, and the gut gets worse. Also, it is quite common for people to drink or smoke more when things get tough, and both these habits are bad for the irritable bowel.

When things are difficult for you, your bowel contracts more than other people's bowels do, causing pain; and this pain is in itself stressful, making a vicious circle of stress-spasm-pain-stress. From now on, your aim must be to break this circle.

There is not much point in taking assorted medicines if you don't tackle the underlying problem – your stress. In fact, if you can recognize that there is a link between stress and your symptoms you will probably benefit more from treatment than if you can't.

There are a few people who cannot accept that their irritable bowel is connected in any way to their personality, or their way of life, or their level of anxiety. They prefer to think it is entirely a physical disease, which they can leave safely in the hands of the doctor – he will prescribe medicines, arrange treatment, and then all will be well. For them, things are unlikely ever to get much better. In the great majority of cases IBS really *is* a stress-related condition, there's no getting away from that, but this doesn't make it any the less real or painful or distressing. (There are, however, some people whose IBS is not related to obvious emotional stress. For them, it may have been triggered by a virus, or by gastro-enteritis, or from some other disease; but even these are conditions that the body finds stressful.)

Finally, why do we feel ashamed or indignant or defensive or apologetic at having a condition that may be caused by stress? It's quite illogical. Do people feel like this because they have coronary heart disease, high blood pressure, colitis, ulcers, or asthma? Yet very often these conditions, which arouse general sympathy, can be caused by stress. Stress will always show itself somewhere, and for you it's in your gut.

So tell yourself 'it's all right to have IBS, it's nothing to feel apologetic or defensive about'. But then add 'however, I'm going to do all I can to reduce the effect it has on me'.

15

What You Can Do About Stress

This chapter is full of ideas for reducing stress, and coping with the stress that you can't get rid of. Some of the ideas may not appeal to you or may not be of any help to you; but some may seem particularly helpful, so work on those. Even if you are not able to remove all the causes, you can at least reduce the more harmful effects.

First of all, learn to recognize signs of stress in yourself. Do you, perhaps, sit on the edge of your chair, or tap your fingers (on the table or the steering wheel), or bang your knees together, or clench your hands or teeth? Do you get a headache, shoulder pains, a sense of restlessness, or fatigue? In all of us, stress shows in one way or another. How does it show itself in you? Think about this, so you can recognize stress the moment it appears.

Next, recognize what it is that causes these stress signals. What makes *you* tense? Your IBS probably comes and goes in response to particular events. Can you recognize in advance that a particular event will trigger it off? Or maybe it doesn't recur until after a stressful event. Could you have known this would happen and done something to prevent it?

Take time to consider what causes IBS to recur for *you*. Perhaps you can now say 'yes, it always gets worse when . . .' If you can do this, you are making progress.

We all have stress, it is inevitable. A small amount can be beneficial, making us perform better, but too much can be really harmful. In your case, stress above a particular level or of a particular type triggers off your irritable bowel. What that level is, only you can tell, but you must now work to keep the stress below the level that triggers IBS for you. How can you do that?

Take pencil and paper, and write down what situations give you the most trouble, which ones you dread most, or get most anxious or agitated about. Then write down why you think this happens. Does your bowel get all irritable in anticipation of these situations, or afterwards? What other physical symptoms do you notice? Write it all down. Your body will remember a stressful situation, so the next time that situation occurs your body will start to produce adrenalin in anticipation of it (it's like our prehistoric friend, Homo Sapiens, on his regular meetings with the greater four-toed mammoth).

Now sit down, look again at that list, and imagine each situation in turn. As you imagine it, see yourself being relaxed in that situation, lower your shoulers, unclench your hands and your jaw, and breathe deeply and evenly until you can think about that situation without anxiety. Do this several times.

It is obvious that you are going to have to make changes. After all if you go on as you are, your IBS will always be there, ready to pounce when things get difficult.

Yet it's never too late to make changes of any sort. Start today. Say to yourself 'as from this very moment I am going to be different in such-and-such a way'. Then stick to it. Nothing dramatic, nothing that you can't keep up, start in a small way, one step at a time. Unless you can do this you'll waste the rest of your life being the way you are now. And it's because you are the way you are that your gut gives you problems.

What follows is a list of ideas, set down at random, any of which may be just right for you. For many of them you will probably say 'well, that's easier said than done; there's no way I can do that'. Only you know whether this is really true, or whether, with a little effort and planning, you could do it if it meant relief from your irritable bowel.

- As you sit at a desk, factory bench, kitchen table, or in the car, bus or train, get into the habit of noticing muscle tension – feet, thighs, abdomen, shoulders, hands, neck, mouth, forehead. And relax. Although you will put aside extra time to relax in peace and quiet, it is important you are also able to relax at any time of day, in a bus queue, traffic jam, office, restaurant, or wherever you are.
- Avoid prolonged driving (which can raise your blood pressure, and get you dreadfully stewed up inside).
- Avoid tight deadlines. It is better to work a longer day without tension than a shorter day with it.
- Have modest goals, both work and personal. Do you really need all that overtime money? Are the things you buy with your money really essential to your inner happiness? Over-ambition can cause great stress to you and your family. Keeping up with the Joneses is not a healthy habit.
- Learn to like people for what they *are*, not for what they *have*. Have as friends people who like you for what you are, not for what you have. After all, you may not always have it.

- Bearing in mind that more stress is caused by things left undone than by things done, be sure to do the things that really matter, so you aren't worrying because you haven't done them.
- Reduce major tasks to manageable components. Plan your time effectively. Divide each day's tasks into priority categories A, B and C. Do the ones marked A, and only if you have time do B and C. If not, leave them. They could be tomorrow's Priority A tasks. There will always be some things that don't get done, so aim to make sure that these are the least important tasks.
- Learn to delegate. Ask your subordinates at work to do something you were going to do, and leave them to get on with it. Ask your children to do some household jobs, and don't keep checking up on them. Even if the job is not done as well or as quickly as you would have done it, does it really matter all that much? A job is hardly ever ruined by being done too slowly.
- Giving and receiving love is a sign of strength, not of weakness. Show physical affection to family and close friends. A hug, or a touch on the arm is a wonderful way of showing you like someone. Have confidence that to touch someone of the same sex does not mean you are gay, and that you can hug someone of the opposite sex without any sexual overtones. Other people do it all the time, so no one will think it odd if you do it, too.
- Develop a hobby that is relaxing and non-competitive. Give time to it.
- Take regular exercise – it lifts the spirits, works off the cares that you get on top of you, revives your outlook on life, gives you more energy, makes it easier to cope with stress. But keep it non-competitive if you can. Squash may keep you fit, but it won't help your irritable bowel one little bit if you worry about your place on the ladder, and are determined to beat everyone you play against. The best forms of exercise are swimming, running, outdoor cycling and brisk walking.
- Pause several times a day to do nothing, to think of pleasant things, to meditate. Read Chapter 19 on meditation, and promise yourself a few minutes a day to yourself. It will do wonders for your gut.
- Stroking the cat is very soothing. Heart specialists often recommend it as a way of reducing blood pressure!
- Try not to have disruptions to too many areas of your life at once. If you are having problems at work, don't stir things up at home. If you have problems at home, try to make sure all is well at work,

and with your friends. If your leisure-time activities are getting you all bothered, keep things calm at home and work.

- Every time something gets you really irritable, or arouses feelings of anger or hostility, write it down *at the time*. Do this every day, and then at the end of the week read what you have been writing down in the preceding days. Do you, perhaps, feel that you have been getting irrationally angry over remarkably trivial things? Do all those things that got you so cross at the time still seem so important several days later?

- We all have a limited ability to withstand stress, and people with IBS possibly have a more limited ability than others. So don't waste the reserves you do have on pointless anger and hostility. If you do, there will be nothing left when you need it. And recognize that anger is not only there when you show it by losing your temper. You may have the sort of nature that keeps things inside you; that doesn't mean you don't feel angry, only that you don't show it outwardly.

- Choose your own goals. Don't necessarily accept the goals set for you by your parents, your spouse, your teacher, your employer. If you fail to live up to goals set by other people this can cause great anxiety.

- Really listen to what other people say. Listen without criticism, without trying to improve on it, without using the word 'I' in your reply. Talking increases blood pressure ever so slightly, and listening decreases it, so spend more time listening than talking, and you will feel calmer.

- Try not to bottle up your emotions. If people take advantage of you, you may find that attending a self-assertiveness course will teach you to express what you feel in a calm, non-threatening way, which will benefit every aspect of your life. Your local library or further education college may have details.

- Most of us like people who make us feel good and increase our self-esteem, and dislike those who make us feel small or incompetent or foolish. What effect do you have on those around you, family, friends, workmates? Think about this very carefully.

- Is your home 'designed for the way you live today'? In other words, is it all planned for people in a hurry? Instant food, microwave oven, breakfast bar where you perch as you bolt your food, fast car that encourages you to rush everywhere, clocks in every room, lots of time-saving gadgets . . . what does this say about the way you live? Slow down. Relax.

- Maintain a balance of work and family time and responsibilities. Try not to let one area of your life dominate the others.
- Share the decision-making; don't take all life's burdens on your shoulders. You'll be amazed how well other people can cope if you trust them to. If someone makes a mistake always give him or her another chance.
- Give your opinions in an honest, loving and non-threatening way.
- If you have problems and anxieties, talk about them. Don't bottle them up. Share your feelings with a friend, and likewise take time to listen to your friend's worries.
- When you know an event is coming which you will find stressful, and which may well trigger your irritable bowel, take extra time for breathing exercises and meditation. Visualize in your mind the stressful event, and see yourself in control and feeling calm about it; work at it until you no longer feel that knot in your stomach.
- Forgive (even if you find it difficult to forget); don't hold grudges. Try to see the situation from the other person's viewpoint and understand why he behaved as he did. If you had been in his shoes might you have done the same thing?
- Anger does more harm to you than it does to the person you are angry with. There's an old Chinese proverb (there always is!) which says: 'Before you seek revenge on your enemy, you must first dig two graves'.
- Stress doesn't just result from pressure from outside – it also results from whether *you* perceive something as being threatening or not. If you have conditioned yourself to regard, say, being overtaken by a woman driver, or having supper served late, as threatening, then every time that happens stress is triggered in you. So rethink what gets you all worked up. Is it really the life-and-death issue you think it is? Do those around you perhaps feel you are making a mountain out of a molehill? They may be right.
- People like people who help people, so see how much you can help others. People also like people whom they help, so receive help willingly and graciously – by making others feel good in themselves, they will feel good towards you.
- Share your feelings, ideas, and frustrations with someone you can trust. If there is no one in your life whom you can trust, why is that? What does it tell you about yourself?
- Have you noticed that the things we complain about in other people are usually the things we ourselves are guilty of?

- Remember that sentence from the Nun's Prayer: 'Teach me the glorious lesson that occasionally I may be mistaken'.
- When you are wrong, apologize. Don't be the sort of person of whom others say 'he just never could admit he was wrong'. If you are not used to it, it is extraordinarily difficult, but it becomes easier with practice, and has a wonderful effect on relationships. Start in a small way 'I'm sorry I spilt the tea', and build up: 'I'm sorry I wasn't here when you wanted me to be'; 'I'm sorry I got cross with you'; 'I'm sorry I didn't give you more of my time'; or even simply 'I'm sorry – I was wrong'.
- Whatever your position in life, consider taking a course in stress management. You will probably learn one or more of the following techniques: to reduce or control the level at which you start to feel angry or anxious, using various forms of relaxation; to recognize what triggers tension in you, and how to prevent it; to change how you look at different situations, so you no longer see them as threatening; not to feel hopeless about your condition.
- At the end of each day, spend time doing relaxation exercises (see Chapter 9). And recall each episode of the day where you felt things got on top of you, or you did not react as well as you would like to have done. Ask yourself 'how could I have handled that better?' Ask yourself whether you have eaten inappropriately, or what has made you feel rushed or stressed; was it necessary and how could you have avoided it? Resolve to make whatever changes will prevent the same thing happening next time.

16
Women and Irritable Bowel Syndrome

If you were to ask the average doctor 'is IBS more common in women or men?', he would almost certainly say 'Oh, it's much more common in women'. It would probably surprise him to know that he is mistaken. IBS affects men and women in roughly equal numbers, with women outnumbering men only slightly. Yet most of the patients he sees with IBS are women; and IBS does seem to affect women differently from men.

Women will probably have first started to get IBS in their twenties and thirties, whereas men typically start rather earlier. Women have headache and backache, as well as the typical IBS symptoms listed in Chapter 1. Whereas men are more likely to get diarrhoea, women more commonly have constipation. This can be particularly troublesome, as women often find an over-full rectum more painful than men do.

Many women notice changes in their bowel habits during the menstrual cycle. This is probably due to hormone changes, and can result in either diarrhoea or constipation. In addition, women often find their irritable bowel is worse during a period, and during sexual intercourse.

Women with undiagnosed IBS are often referred to a gynaecological clinic, where their pain will be discussed but their bowel habits are probably not investigated. This simply delays the correct diagnosis. Up to one-third of all women with IBS have had some sort of gynaecological operation in an attempt to solve their stomach pain, and, of course, as the pain is due to an irritable bowel rather than some other cause, the problem is usually just as bad after the operation as it was before. (The equivalent operation for men will probably be removal of the appendix, and it is equally unlikely to cure the problem.)

The working woman, whatever her job, has particular stresses. Women often do more monotonous boring jobs than men, and boredom – whether at work or from being 'just a housewife' – is stressful. If she is a high-powered executive she may feel guilty and selfish asserting her wishes, in contrast with men in the same position who tend to thrive on exerting power and control. She may feel she has to work harder and more effectively than her male colleagues just to hang on to her job. If, in addition to this, a woman has a husband and children, she may feel additional guilt at neglecting her traditional role as home-maker, as well as stress when she doesn't neglect it and tries to fulfil several roles at once.

Most books on stress are written with men in mind, usually highly-stressed businessmen. And so the solutions are more geared to men than to women. Yet women have just as much stress as men (albeit of a different kind), and just as many stress-related diseases, but neither the women themselves nor their doctors seem to take them as seriously. Whereas a man might have lots of tests and is then told to have a complete rest, women are more likely to be prescribed tranquillisers and told 'don't worry, relax, it's nothing a good night's sleep won't cure'.

Most women have come across the condescending attitude of some (particularly older) male doctors – 'don't be silly, dear lady', 'we have got a vivid imagination, haven't we?', 'you really do ask too many questions, my dear'. If you have a doctor like this, you might be more at ease with a younger doctor, or with a woman doctor.

Doctors are not God. They are just ordinary fallible people like you and me. You have every right to regard them as your equals, to ask them questions and expect courteous answers, and to receive from them as much respect as you give them.

Stress among women is also caused by being too anxious to please, or being afraid to displease, or by putting up with unfair or unpleasant situations.

For example, a working husband may spend his lunch hour having a leisurely meal, possibly in the pub with 'the boys', drive home in the car at the end of the day, put his feet up for a while when he gets home, and then spend the evening watching television, going out to the pub, or doing whatever *he* wants to do. Children, if he has them, probably make very little difference to this routine.

In contrast, his working wife spends her lunch hour shopping and queuing, comes home on public transport laden with bags, sets to and gets the supper, may have to entertain her husband's boss, and probably wade through a pile of ironing before bedtime. If she has children she may have to accept a less interesting job because it fits in with school hours, and it is she who is expected to take time off work if they are ill. It is also the grown-up daughter who generally looks after elderly parents.

And let us think a minute about family holidays. Does the

husband spend his holiday answering the phone, working on a production line, attending business meetings, and all the things he does during a normal working day? Certainly not! Yet each year millions of wives take self-catering 'holidays', where they do exactly what they do at home – shop, cook, clean, iron – only in much less suitable surroundings. At the end of the fortnight, I wonder who returns the more rested!

At work women are likely to have more boring jobs than men, to have to cope with sexism, male chauvinism, low pay, and such attitudes as 'don't you worry your pretty little head about that'.

Not content with all this, we really are experts in feelings of guilt and self-reproach. Given half a chance we women will feel guilty either because we *don't* work, don't contribute financially, have 'a meal ticket for life', and fill the day doing trivial things; or because we *do* work, are not at home being a 'home-maker', don't give husband and children as much time as we should, and perhaps sometimes we would honestly rather be at work than at home. We are wonderful at feeling guilty if we dare to relax, don't do something we ought to have done, and fall short of the ideals we set for ourselves.

So what can you, a young woman, an older woman, a woman with husband and children or without, do about all this? After all, the more you can make some changes, the more likely you are to keep your irritable bowel under control.

- Write down on paper all the things that cause you stress. Then decide which ones can be changed by some action on your part, and which you must accept and learn to live with. The more you can get rid of, the more inner resources you will have left to cope with the rest. You probably know the saying by Reinhold Niebuhr: 'grant me the serenity to accept the things I cannot change, the courage to change the things I can, and the wisdom to know the difference'. So let's have plenty of serenity and courage.
- From today onwards accept that it's OK to relax, to make some space for yourself. Give yourself permission to take time off, to fall short of your ideals, and to make changes at work or at home that will allow this. Decide from today onwards that it's quite all right to be a working mother, or an assertive career woman, or a stay-at-home wife, or whatever role you see yourself in.
- Be good to yourself. You are entitled to as much rest, recreation, and personal space as everyone else. Using your most non-aggressive manner, let other people realize this.

- If you have children, encourage them to cook, iron their clothes, do the washing up, put the family's clothes away, etc. Enjoy the fact that they are doing it, thank them, and don't worry that it might not be done as well as you would have done it.
- See if you can persuade your husband to share the domesticity; it may be unrealistic to hope that he will clean the toilet, but perhaps he can share the ironing, shopping, and cooking? Is he no good at cooking? Well perhaps you weren't that good at it when you got married, and you just had to learn; couldn't he learn, too?
- Try to establish a routine where everyone shares the domestic duties. Or have you, perhaps, built up your own little Empire where no one else feels able, capable or welcome to do these things, and then do you wonder why you are left to do it all while they watch television, play football, or go out?
- At work, is it you who gets lumbered with the coffee-making, washing up, popping out for biscuits, etc., just because you are a woman? If you have a job that is of similar importance to a man's, try to get the men to do some of these jobs. Instead of the men saying 'Jane, sweetie, just pop out and get me some cigarettes, there's a pet', see if you can get them to say 'Jane, I'm going out for some cigarettes, can I get you anything?'
- If your IBS gets worse around the time of your periods, be sure to do relaxation exercises then.
- When you do take time off, enjoy it. There's no need to offer excuses to everyone, simply a quiet explanation. Don't spoil this time by feeling guilty about it. Nor should you expect those around you to feel annoyed with you – they almost certainly won't, unless you become so guilty and defensive it provokes them into annoyance.
- Indulge yourself sometimes, without feeling that self-indulgence is bad.
- When you feel 'I *really* should . . .', say 'it's all right not to'.
- Learn first aid and basic home health management, so you don't worry or panic about illness and accidents. Learn how to mend a fuse, change a plug, change a tyre, put up a shelf, turn off the electricity and mains water, and similar things so you are not dependent on other people who may not be there when you need them. Make sure you understand the family finances, so you don't fear being left alone to cope.

17
Take a Good Look At Yourself

Have you ever wondered whether there might be a connection between your irritable bowel and the sort of person you are? It has long been recognized by general practitioners that certain diseases are often found in people with certain types of personality – maybe IBS is one of them. You might have talked to other people with this condition and felt that, in many ways, you have a lot in common.

It seems that people with IBS are likely to belong to one of two personality types. Those belonging to the first type

- are strong, forceful and aggressive
- are competitive and keen to win
- fill every moment of their time
- have a great wish to achieve something
- use their energy and drive to benefit others
- motivate other people, often for good
- are conscientious and hardworking
- may become easily annoyed or angry
- have a fast emphatic way of speaking
- often use obscenities or bad language
- are very conscious of time
- go 'all out' when they tackle something.

Those belonging to the second type

- find it difficult to say 'no'
- are perfectionists and hardworking
- are seldom satisfied with their achievements
- keep their feelings bottled up inside them
- are afraid to show anger and hostility
- may be impatient and irritable
- may often be taken advantage of by other people.

If you feel the first category sums you up quite well, ask yourself whether being like this keeps you in a state of constant activity and tension, causing your body to produce a lot of adrenalin, and therefore contributing directly to your irritable bowel. If so, some of the following ideas may help you:

74

- Do one thing at a time. Decide that as from today you will not: telephone or shave while driving, telephone while doing the ironing, watch TV while preparing notes for tomorrow, mark homework while cooking supper, or whatever particular combination of things you do.
- Cut out all obscenities and bad language from your speech. Perhaps you use them because they give you extra weight or to express anger and violence. But they seldom reduce hostility, and frequently intensify it. If you listen to other people's speech that is full of obscenities, wouldn't you agree that it sounds rather ugly?
- Don't call other people by insulting names. Not only does it wind you up, it also makes you seem an unpleasant person.
- Play to lose sometimes, especially with children; don't worry about your golf handicap or your position on the squash ladder. Learn to play simply for the fun of it, without a sense of competitiveness.
- Drive in the slow lane; don't keep trying to overtake. If you are late, resolve that tomorrow you will leave earlier so that you can drive more slowly and courteously. It will also do wonders for your blood pressure.
- One day, at a suitable time, record yourself having a longish conversation with someone. Play it back when you are on your own, and notice if you talk too quickly, interrupt frequently, sound hurried or opinionated, or start speaking before the other person has completely finished.
- Wear a watch as seldom as possible. If you must wear one, put a red dot on it to remind yourself not to look at it so often.
- Perhaps in the past you have quickly forgotten what other people have told you about themselves or their families; this may cause them to think you are uninterested and uncaring. So, next time you make social conversation with someone you don't know particularly well, decide that by the end of it you will know more about him and his life and interests than he will about yours. This involves listening more than talking. Next time you see him, recall what he told you, and enquire about him. He will really appreciate it.
- The more you can listen to other people, the more you gain their respect and liking. After all, don't we all like people who bother to listen to us, and have less liking for those who never listen and always talk?

- Pay attention to the things worth *being*, rather than the things worth *having*.
- Avoid getting annoyed or angry about things that don't annoy or anger calmer people. How often is it worth losing your temper?
- Remember that a job is hardly ever ruined by being done too slowly.
- If you are going to make changes to the way you do things, try telling this to someone you can trust, someone who will not belittle you. Often, just telling someone gives you a greater will to see it through. Even if you can't do this, the fact that you have decided to make changes means the battle is half won.
- Enjoy beautiful things that have no monetary value – a spider's web, a bird building its nest, children playing happily, old people talking together.
- Twice a day, make a point of listening to someone talking to you without interrupting at all.
- Try learning yoga. It is non-competitive and non-judgemental, and you will surely enjoy the sense of harmony it brings you. If possible join a class, but if you can't do that, a good book for beginners, which may be available from your local library, is *Yoga* by Sophy Hoare, published by Macdonald Guidelines in 1977.
- Harness your drive, sense of purpose and enthusiasm to work for good.
- Avoid confrontation with other strong-minded individuals. F. Scott Fitzgerald said 'Very strong personalities must confine themselves in mutual conversations to very gentle subjects'.

You may, however, feel that the second category sums up your personality rather better. If so, some of these ideas may help you:

- Put aside time each day (or a longer period each week if that is easier) that it is entirely *your* time. Use it to do whatever you want to do, without any sense of guilt. Allow yourself to enjoy doing things of your choice in that time. If you think 'I *really* ought to do such-and-such', then *don't* do it. This time is not for things that you *ought* to do, but for things that you *want* to do. If your life is so rushed that you cannot find time for yourself, then make some changes. It may involve getting up a bit earlier, or giving something up, or doing a tedious chore rather less often; do whatever you can to find time for yourself.

- Try learning to say 'no'. As you lie in the bath, or sit quietly on your own, visualize a situation in which someone is going to ask you to do something you don't really want to do. And then visualize yourself saying a polite but firm 'no'. Think up a form of words that sounds right to you, that won't put the other person's back up, and then say them several times. Go over this in your mind several times, until you are comfortable with the result. Then when it happens 'for real', you will find it easier to say 'no'.
- Perhaps there is someone in your life to whom you just never can say 'no'. It may be your boss, or your husband, or someone else. Every time he asks something of you, you automatically say 'yes'. All right then, imagine he has asked you to do something dreadful, like murder someone. Would you say 'Yes'? 'No, of course I wouldn't.' Fine, you have now accepted that there is a situation in which you are capable of saying 'no' to that person. So build on that. Imagine other situations in which you know for certain that you would say 'no'. In your mind practise saying 'no'. Then visualize less extreme circumstances, and again visualize yourself saying 'no'. Then perhaps quite ordinary circumstances, and again visualise yourself saying 'no'. The more you practise it, the easier it will become.
- There is, after all, no one so trodden on as a human doormat. The more you just lie there, letting everyone take advantage of you, the more they will go on doing it. It won't occur to them to do anything different. But once you have said 'no' a few times, politely but firmly, they will quickly realize that you are not a doormat, and eventually they will treat you with the consideration you deserve. Realise that you are put upon because you let yourself be. So resolve that, from today onwards, things are going to be different.
- Accept other people's bad behaviour towards you. If you can accept that they just are the way they are, then when they behave badly towards you it will be no more than you expected anyway, and so you won't feel too badly about it. If you keep hoping unrealistically that a particular person will one day undergo a magical change and treat you quite differently, you will become unhappy, frustrated, and angry. Be able to forgive, but that doesn't mean you have to give in all the time.
- On a piece of paper, make a list of your good points. Don't feel embarrassed about doing this, just delight in the pleasant side of your nature.

- Many people with IBS have a suppressed inner anger – if you keep your anger cooped up, as in a pressure cooker, one day it will all come bursting out in a way that will probably cause great hurt to you and to people you care about. So learn to express your anger non-aggressively, and don't bottle it up.
- Anger makes you frustrated, prevents you from finding rational solutions to your problems, and can make you ill. My earlier book, *Sleep Like a Dream – The Drug-free Way*, published by Sheldon Press, has lots of practicable ideas for reducing anger.

18

Irritable Bowel Syndrome and Your Family

Is irritable bowel syndrome hereditary? Probably not. Can it run in families? Yes.

This may seem contradictory! 'Hereditary' means it is inherited genetically from your ancestors, and that there is very little you can do to prevent yourself getting it. Current evidence suggests heredity plays only a minor part in IBS. For example, it is much more common in first-borns than in others, and if it were strongly hereditary it would occur more evenly among all the children of a family.

There are, however, several reasons why it might run in families. Firstly, members of the same family may have the same sort of personality, and this personality may increase their tendency to stress. Secondly, members of the same family may have the same sort of diet, and this may increase the chance that they will all be, say, constipated. Thirdly, members of the same family may treat that constipation in the same way – wrongly.

Let us suppose that your elderly great-aunts were permanently constipated (though I don't suppose this was ever something they talked about!). This might have been because they took very little exercise, ate a bland diet with no dietary fibre, and took regular doses of liquid paraffin or other purgatives every day 'for regularity'. So this constipation was not something that they had inherited, or passed on to you. It was directly linked to their way of life.

If your father had IBS, could this be because he was often under a lot of stress? Never relaxed? Ate very little dietary fibre? And picked it up after a bout of 'holiday tummy'?

So a shared physical and emotional environment is more likely to account for the fact that some of your close relatives may have IBS than is heredity. That said, there are two factors which may run in families. One is intolerance to dairy products caused by an enzyme deficiency, and the other is an abnormality of the smooth muscle of the colon. Both these may be present with IBS, and both may be hereditary.

'Indigestion' problems often start in infancy. The colicky baby may become a constipated child, frequently complaining of tummy ache. As a young teenager he may have irregular bowel habits, still with occasional tummy ache. By the time he is in his late teens or early twenties he may even have had an operation to try to get to the bottom of it. But if the cause was IBS, removing his appendix is not going to solve the problem!

A survey in London found that children with recurring abdominal pain often came from families with a similar problem. In addition, members of their families had had more operations than usual, and visited the doctor more often. The families concerned tended to have more marriage breakdowns and other forms of stress than other families. Think carefully about whether your family life may cause stomach problems in your children, because about one-third of adults with IBS have had the symptoms since childhood.

Quite a lot of research has been done into how people with IBS were treated as children, to see if past history offers any clues to present problems. Probably the most interesting finding is that, as children, they were more likely to be allowed to stay off school if they had stomach ache than if they had other disorders, like headaches. Also if they had stomach ache they were often given gifts or special food, but not when they had other complaints. It is easy to see how a child can quickly associate stomach ache with parental sympathy, with gifts and with days off school.

Of course, none of this may apply to you. Your IBS may have appeared for the first time in adulthood. But if you have IBS, then there is a chance that it may be in part due to the way you were brought up; also it is possible that your son or daughter may get it, because of the sort of physical and emotional household that he or she has been brought up in. It might therefore be worth your while looking at the way you bring up your children, to see if you are forming habits now that may cause IBS later.

If your child has persistent tummy ache, get it properly diagnosed by a doctor. After all, the outlook is better if it is caught early. If the diagnosis is IBS, you can help your child greatly in the following ways:

- Allow her time and space to visit the toilet in peace and without embarrassing comments about noise, smell, and the time she takes.
- Because children and young people are so easily put off using the toilet, make yours as attractive as possible – carpet, curtains, interesting things on the wall, a shelf of books and magazines, or a radio or cassette player.

- Be aware if she is feeling anxious about anything, and take it seriously without turning it into a momentous world issue.
- Teach her simple methods of relaxation.
- Make sure she eats healthy meals, with plenty of dietary fibre, and without feeling rushed.
- Establish a good routine at the start of the day, allowing time for a wholesome leisurely breakfast, and time to establish regular bowel habits.
- Allow her to feel able to discuss bowel habits with you without embarrassment, yet at the same time keeping the subject low-key so that she doesn't become obsessive about it.
- If she complains of persistent tummy ache, get it checked by the doctor, but don't reward her, or make her tummy ache a constant subject of discussion.

These are ways directly related to IBS in which you can help. But there are other ways, too. The ideas that follow are taken from various sources, including several pieces of research on IBS personality, and I list them without any sense of being holier-than-thou. Bringing up children is difficult, but, you may believe, as I do, that helping to build the generation that follows us is one of the most important (and undervalued) jobs in the world. If you can follow most of these ideas you will have children you can find joy in –and they probably won't have IBS!

- Bearing in mind that many people with IBS have had a series of events in their lives that cause stress and hopelessness leading to anxiety, do all you can to make sure this does not happen to your children.
- Show love openly to your adolescent children, and thus help them to grow into loving adults.
- Really listen to what your children say. Then say something encouraging, not something instructive, or competitive, or that makes them feel small.
- Many children believe they are loved only if they are winners. So praise your children for the effort they make, not just for achievement. Make them feel proud of whatever they achieve, however small it seems to you.
- Help them find their own solutions to problems. Don't force your views on them. In discussion see how seldom you can use the word 'I'.

- Cut down on the verbal advice. Instead, uphold by your own conduct the sort of person you would like your son or daughter to become. Most children model themselves on their parents for much of their childhood.
- Some hard-driving parents never let their children win at family games, because they believe this instils the right competitive attitude for life. But it can produce a child who grows into an angry adult, always driving for achievement. Introduce your child to sport without leagues and trophies to be constantly striving for.
- When you play games with your children, end each session at a point of confidence and success, don't continue to exhaustion or failure.
- Many parents cannot stand being corrected, or criticized or disagreed with by their children. Practise saying to your children 'yes, you're right about that, and I'm wrong'.
- Encourage them to express their emotions. Even boys can cry.
- Allow children to make mistakes; in recovering from these mistakes they gain self-confidence.
- Don't insist on perfect behaviour all the time – life will be much more peaceful.
- Never hit your children. If you hit them a lot you will quite probably turn them into aggressive adults, with your sons growing into violent men who hit their wives and children, and your daughters growing into depressive women who find it difficult to show love to their children. And so the cycle continues.
- Keep in mind this quotation from Goethe: 'We can't form our children on our own concepts; we must take them and love them as God gives them to us.'
- Or this from Kahlil Gibran: 'You may give them your love but not your thoughts, for they have their own thoughts. You may house their bodies but not their souls, for their souls dwell in the house of tomorrow, which you cannot visit, not even in your dreams. You may strive to be like them, but seek not to make them like you, for life goes not backward nor tarries with yesterday.'

19

Learn To Relax

Relaxation

Doctors' and research workers' acceptance that relaxation can be very effective in reducing all manner of illness has been well documented in learned journals. Yet despite the well-publicized hazards of tranquillisers, and the number of stress-related problems that their patients bring them every day, doctors still spend more time prescribing tranquillisers than teaching or recommending relaxation. This is quite understandable, given the limited resources of time and money that a busy doctor can spend on each patient, and the fact that most doctors see themselves as doctors and not teachers of relaxation. Yet time taken to learn relaxation and stress-reduction techniques would result in fewer stress-related diseases, less time off work, less domestic tension, less burden on doctors – and thus benefit everyone.

All the techniques in this chapter are different ways of achieving the same end – a state of peaceful relaxation and contentment. A quiet mind will lead to a quiet stomach. You may find one method appeals to you more than another; if so, then work at it until its benefits improve your general well-being, and, hopefully, your irritable bowel.

The environment you choose for your relaxation exercises (or meditation) should be quiet, at a comfortable temperature, with no distractions and no sense of urgency. Whether to sit or lie down is up to you – there is no 'right' way. If you sit, choose a low chair, and sit with your feet flat on the floor, your spine straight, and imagine that the crown of your head is being gently pulled upwards by a thread, straightening your spine as it does so. If you lie down, the ideal surface is a blanket on a carpeted floor (a bed is usually too soft); lie on your back with small cushions under your neck and knees, or with your knees slightly flexed. The main thing is that you should be comfortable.

Try the following exercises. At first nothing may seem to happen, you may be disappointed, and feel this is for other people but not for you. Take heart, don't give up. Regular relaxation (and meditation) will do you good, even if you are unaware of it. Some people give up when they don't see instant results, but this is a pity because benefits begin before you are aware of any improvement.

At the end of each exercise remain quietly for a few minutes, then stretch from your heels to your fingertips, and if you are lying down roll over on to your side for a few minutes. Then open your eyes, bring your awareness back to the present, and when you are ready get up.

Exercise 1. Lie in the yoga Corpse Pose for about 10 minutes a day, thus: take off your shoes, loosen belts, remove glasses if you wear them, and lie on your back with your feet 1–2 feet (30–60 cm) apart, arms slightly away from your sides with palms facing upwards. Allow your feet to roll comfortably outwards. Move as necessary until you feel symmetrical. Then close your eyes and just relax. Breathe through your nose and notice your abdomen rising and falling with each breath. Try to keep your mind empty of all troubling thoughts; if this is difficult, choose one of the breathing or meditation exercises that will help you to concentrate on the here and now.

Exercise 2. Sit or lie comfortably. Focus your thoughts on your abdomen, and slowly tense the abdominal muscles. Then relax them. Imagine warmth and tranquillity flowing over the whole bowel area. Be aware of any tension in this region, and make a conscious effort to overcome it.

Exercise 3. As you sit or lie quietly, turn your thoughts to each part of your body in turn – your feet, legs, buttocks, abdomen, chest, hands, arms, neck, jaw, mouth, nose, eyes, forehead. As you think about each part of you, tense that part up. Then increase the tension. Now relax. Work upwards from your feet to your head, tensing and relaxing, concentrating especially on any part of you that you often tense up. Eventually your whole body will be beautifully relaxed.

Exercise 4. As Exercise 3, but instead of tensing each part of your body, concentrate on it and say 'my [right foot] is warm and soft and heavy'. Imagine that foot sinking deeply into the floor, so heavy that you couldn't possibly lift it up. Continue upwards from your feet to your head, until each part of you feels deliciously warm and soft and heavy.

In addition, any of the following can help you to relax:

- Buy a cassette tape of relaxation or 'mood' music – ask at a record shop, or health-food shop, or look in the advertisements in magazines such as *Yoga Today* or *Here's Health*.
- Drink a relaxing herb tea. Try one containing camomile or valerian.
- Have a warm (not too hot) bath, with soothing additives such as camomile, valerian or sandalwood oil.
- Sit in a chair in front of a long mirror. How do you look? Tense, or relaxed? Are you sitting on the edge of the chair, or comfortably back into it? What are your hands doing? Practise sitting in a way that, seen in the mirror, looks relaxed and at peace. Then take your new-found knowledge, and use it every time you sit in a chair. This will help you to see yourself as others see you.
- Or, as you go about the house, stop, and without changing your facial expression, look at yourself in the mirror. What do you see? What do others see? A frown, a tight mouth, or a calm pleasant facial expression? Relax your face, smile at yourself in the mirror.
- It is true that you cannot have a relaxed body with a tense mind, so obviously you must calm your mind before you can calm your body. But, to a limited extent, you can put the cart before the horse. By making your body relaxed, you can indeed start to relax your mind. So make sure that each part of you is without tension, outwardly still, and you will be a long way towards making yourself inwardly still.

Meditation

If you have IBS, it is quite possible you also have high blood pressure, a fast pulse, and a high level of anxiety or tension. If so, meditation may be just the thing for you. It lowers heartbeat and blood pressure, decreases anxiety, gives a feeling of calm, relaxation, relief from tension, and better sleep; it also increases alertness, ability to concentrate and general well-being. With all that going for it, why not give it a try?

People who practise meditation regularly are less anxious than others, less prone to stress, and recover quicker after stressful incidents. To describe the effects of meditation on them, they use words such as 'an inner quietness', 'peace', 'pleasant feelings', 'contentment', 'relaxation', 'calmness'. It sounds good, doesn't it?

As with breathing exercises, self-hypnosis and relaxation, meditation should be practised regularly. Ten to twenty minutes a day is ideal. Choose a time of day when you won't be tired, or liable to interruption. Find a quiet comfortable place. If you can do it at the same time and in the same place every day you will find it more beneficial, but don't worry if you can't.

Sit comfortably with your spine straight, on a chair with your feet flat on the ground, or on a cushion on the floor, or on a meditation stool if you have one. Close your eyes and take several slow deep breaths. Be aware of any tensions in your mind, or in your body. Notice them, and try to overcome them.

There is no 'correct' response to meditation, or to relaxation exercises. Your mind and body will respond in their own way. Don't try to force things, just be patient and passive, and with time you will be pleased at the changes you start to notice, both in your mind and, hopefully, in your irritable bowel.

In meditation it is important to divert your mind from your normal thought processes. Suspend all judgement. Don't be critical. Just notice what is happening without thinking about it intellectually.

As a beginner, meditating may bring thoughts to the surface of your mind that make you feel agitated or anxious. This is quite normal. We all have things buried deep in our minds that we would prefer not to think about, but as a general rule these thoughts are better out than in. So recognize them, try not to let yourself become distressed by them, and gradually they will no longer affect you.

Here are some simple exercises in meditation. Try each one several times, and see which works best for you. Don't expect instant results, neither should you dismiss it as a load of rubbish. Practise it every day, and you will learn to achieve a calm state of mind.

Exercise 1. Close your eyes. Be aware of relaxing all your muscles in turn from your feet up to your head. Concentrate particularly on whatever part of your body you often tense up. It could be your abdomen, shoulders, hands, neck, mouth, forehead. Consciously relax that part. Breathe through your nose, and notice your normal regular breathing. After a few moments, as you breathe out say the word 'one' either out loud or to yourself.

Then breathe in normally. Continue like this, saying 'one' each time you breathe out. Try to concentrate on the normal breathing and the word 'one'. Your mind will probably wander, and if it does just be aware of this and bring your thoughts gently back to the word 'one'. After about 10 minutes continue normal breathing without saying 'one', just sitting quietly for a while with your eyes closed. Then open your eyes, and sit for a few minutes in the same position. When you are ready, stand up. Don't worry whether you have successfully achieved deep relaxation; it will come in its own time.

Exercise 2. Close your eyes and breathe rhythmically and normally through your nose for two or three minutes, noticing the breath enter and leave the body. Now focus on your exhalation. Notice the warmth of the breath in your nostrils. Each time you breathe out think the word 'relax' (or 'peace', or whatever word seems right for you). Feel your body sinking, feeling warm and slow. Be aware of letting go a little bit more with each breath. Each time you exhale imagine the tension leaving your body with the breath. Continue like this for as long as you wish.

Exercise 3. As you breathe normally, focus on the rise and fall of your abdomen, and of the air flowing in and out of your nostrils. As you breathe *in* count 1, and as you breathe *out* count 2, *in* count 3, *out* count 4, and so on up to 10. Then start again: *in* 1, *out* 2, *in* 3, *out* 4 . . . Don't attempt to control or manipulate your breath. Just let it happen naturally, being aware of it. Notice if your mind wanders, and bring your thoughts gently back to your breath, and to the rising and falling of your abdomen. Repeat as many times as you wish.

Exercise 4. Place a lighted candle a few feet in front of you. Concentrate on it until you feel you can't look at it any longer. Then shut your eyes, and you will see the after-image of the candle and the flame in front of you. Concentrate on this after-image until it fades from your mind. Then open your eyes and look at the real candle again. Repeat this as many times as you wish.

Exercise 5. Hold any beautiful object in your hands, and examine it most thoroughly. Think about it as much as you can. Don't think about anything else. If, for example, you are holding a leaf, look at the veins, the patterns they form, the colours; think about the life cycle that produced that leaf – seed, plant. fruits – and of the wild insects or creatures for whom that leaf is important. Spend time enjoying its beauty. Or perhaps you are holding a piece of pottery; if so feel its shape, its texture; think about its colour, and about its transformation from a lump of raw clay. Concentrate on these things of beauty, and don't allow your mind to wander to your present problems.

Exercise 6. Hold five beads or pebbles in one hand. Pass them slowly one at a time to the other hand. Feel each one, count it, hear the sound it makes against the others. Focus your attention on the beads. Repeat this, passing the beads from one hand to the other many times.

Exercise 7. Close your eyes, and transport your mind to a place you remember that was peaceful and relaxing. Imagine yourself there, notice the sights, sounds and smells with pleasure and enjoyment. Sense the peacefulness, the feeling of refreshment. After a few minutes open your eyes and stretch. Realize that you can return in your mind to that place whenever you want to feel calm. (Be sure to choose somewhere that produces no unpleasant thoughts. If you can't find somewhere like that, what does that say about you, your personality, the sort of conflicts you generate during your life?)

When you have finished meditating, stay quietly in the same position for a few minutes. Then stretch from your heels to your fingertips, open your eyes, return your awareness to your present surroundings, and when you are ready get up.

Breathing exercises

Since IBS tends to get worse when you are under stress, and probably gets better when you feel calm, it follows that the more you can do to have a quiet mind the more likely you are to have a quiet stomach.

One of the easiest ways to feel calm and relaxed is to do breathing exercises. These are not 'way out', 'weird', or 'hippy'. They are used by ordinary people, by high-powered executives, low-powered non-executives, housewives, students, by people just like you and me, as a means to feel inwardly quiet and tranquil. You can do them anywhere and at any time.

If you have never tried breathing exercises before, you must start in the right frame of mind. Don't say to yourself 'this is all a load of rubbish and I know it won't work'. Neither should you expect instant success. Take your time, be prepared to have several sessions before you sense any improvement. Try to feel positive and enthusiastic about doing it.

Although you can indeed do them anywhere and at any time, it will probably be most helpful if you can choose a place that is quiet and a time that is unhurried. Lots of people get most help by doing them as soon as they get up, before the busy-ness of the day begins. Maybe for you a few quiet minutes in a lunch hour would be right; and if you do them at bedtime you will almost certainly sleep really well.

So, you are in a quiet room and it is a quiet time. Sit in an upright chair, with your spine straight, and the crown of your head feeling as if it is being gently pulled up like a puppet on a string. (The crown is a lot further back than the forehead.) Place your feet flat on the floor, and rest your hands comfortably on your thighs or on your lap. Remove your glasses if you wear them, and your shoes if you want to.

Choose one of these exercises, and do it for at least 10 minutes. You may look at your watch when you think the time is nearly up, but don't set an alarm.

If you are not used to doing breathing exercises, you may find, as with meditation, that thoughts come to the surface of your mind that have been buried for a long time, and these thoughts may be upsetting. If this happens, accept them, be aware of them, and try not to become agitated by them. Most thoughts of this kind are better out than in.

Breathing exercises have the apparently contradictory effect of giving you energy when you feel tired, and calming you down when you feel tense. So, whether you feel tired or tense, don't have a cigarette, a cup of coffee, or an alcoholic drink – nicotine, caffeine and alcohol can all aggravate your irritable bowel; instead, just breathe deeply for a minute or so.

Whenever you find yourself in a difficult or stressful situation, take a few deep breaths, lower your shoulders, unclench your hands and your jaw, work consciously to slow down that beating heart and racing breath. Try to think with compassion and understanding of the situation. After all, getting all stewed up will simply make your irritable bowel worse, and now at least you know *you* can do something about it.

Most of the breathing exercises which follow are taken from my earlier book *Sleep Like a Dream – The Drug-free Way*, published by Sheldon Press.

Breathing exercise 1

Sit quietly, hands resting in your lap, spine straight, with no feeling of tension. Breathe deeply and slowly. As you breathe in, think 'calm in', and see in your mind a great river of calm flowing into your body with each incoming breath. As you breathe out, think 'stress out', and really imagine all the stress, anger, pain and tension flowing out of your body with each outgoing breath. Concentrate totally on the breathing, and if your mind wanders bring it gently back to your inward and outward breath.

Breathing exercise 2 (Alternate Nostril)

Firstly, the naming of parts: in order to identify your fingers correctly, working outwards from the thumb, they are the thumb, index finger, middle finger, ring finger, little finger.

Sit with your spine straight, eyes shut, and all your body relaxed. If you wear glasses it is best to remove them. (1) Place index and middle fingers of right hand on bridge of nose between eyebrows, and with the palm of your hand facing towards your nose. (2) With ring finger of right hand close the left nostril. (Reverse instructions if you prefer to use your left hand.) (3) Breathe *out* through right nostril, then breathe *in* through right nostril. (4) Lift ring finger slightly and close right nostril with thumb, breathe *out* through left nostril, then *in* through left nostril. (5) Lift thumb slightly and repeat from (2) for several minutes, remembering to breathe *out* first through each nostril. Listen to your breathing. Concentrate on it. If your mind wanders, be aware of this, and bring it gently back.

This exercise sounds complicated to describe, but once you see how to do it, it is a simple soothing rhythm. Gentle pressure on the nostrils is thought to relieve menstrual cramps, so there is a possibility that it might relieve abdominal cramps too.

Breathing exercise 3 (Solar Plexus)

Do this exercise when you wake up, and at bedtime. Lie on the bed. Place hands on your solar plexus, just below the base of the ribs, with fingertips touching. Breathe *out* deeply. Pause. Breathe *in* slowly through the nose, feeling your fingertips separate. Pause. Breathe *out* slowly, feeling your fingertips come together. Continue this slow, calm, deep breathing, and concentrate on your breath. If your mind wanders, be aware of it, and bring it gently back to the breath.

Variation of exercise 3

Instead of pausing, breathe in and out in one complete circular movement.

Breathing exercise 4

1. Breathe *out* deeply to get rid of stale air.
2. Breathe *in* slowly and deeply to count of *two*.
3. Hold breath for a count of *four*.
4. Breathe *out* for a count of *four*.

i.e. *in* two – *hold* four – *out* four. Do this for two or three minutes, but stop if you feel dizzy. If you have high blood pressure hold your breath for a count of two, not four.

Breathing exercise 5

Open your mouth slightly, and breathe in and out through your nose and mouth at the same time.

Breathing exercise 6 (Exhale)

1. Breathe *in* normally.
2. Breathe *out* for as long as you can.
3. Breathe *in* normally.
4. Breathe *out* normally.

Continue this sequence for as long as you like.

Exercise 7 is one to be done when you have tried at least one or more of the others several times. Its purpose is to show you that you can control how your body works, and use this control to your advantage. It is in three parts:

First, spend some minutes doing one of the earlier breathing exercises, and achieving a state of calm. Notice how your heart is beating quite slowly and evenly, that your abdomen is rising slowly and regularly as you breathe from low down in your lungs. This is a pleasant relaxed state, and if you could exist like this most of the time you would very seldom have an irritable bowel.

Next, recall an experience that arouses hostile feelings in you – perhaps a recent argument, or a sense of injustice done to you, or something that causes you to feel angry. It may be a row with your spouse or someone at work, or a disagreement with another driver or a neighbour, or whatever has angered you. Go over it in your mind for a few minutes. Now notice how, as your mind becomes churned up, your body does too. Your heart may be beating quite fast, you may be sweating slightly, you may clench your teeth or your hands, and I expect you are breathing quickly and from high up in your lungs, so that your upper chest rises and falls rapidly.

At this stage, pause. Recognize what is happening to you. Can you accept that what goes on in your mind has a clear, noticeable, and rather unpleasant effect on your body? Most people with chronic IBS have a faster pulse than average, and often they have high blood pressure too. They breathe from high up in their lungs. These are all typical signs of a stressed body, and here you have proved to yourself that, having been in a state of relaxation, you have now reproduced these 'stress' signs in your body simply by thinking stressful thoughts.

Then try to get your body back into the state it was in before you churned it up. Put the unpleasant thoughts out of your mind, and replace them with thoughts that give you joy and pleasure. Do one of the breathing or meditation exercises that makes you think of something else. Do it for as long as it takes for your heartbeat to slow down, your breathing to become quiet and regular, and for that feeling of calm to descend again. Be aware that you *can* do it by yourself. You really don't need cigarettes, alcohol or tranquillisers to induce relaxation. By using even simple breathing exercises you can change a state of stress into a state of calm.

There must surely be a lesson in this for people with irritable bowel syndrome.

20

Alternative Medicine – an Introduction

'Man's body and mind, with the utmost reverence to both I speak it, are exactly like a jerkin and a jerkin's lining; rumple the one and you rumple the other.' Laurence Sterne, *Tristram Shandy*.

If irritable bowel syndrome has been troubling you for, say, two years or more, you may be finding that the conventional medical treatment of anti-spasmodics, bulk laxatives and perhaps a mild anti-depressant is not working all that well. This approach is, after all, just treating the symptoms without tackling the underlying cause. Have you considered alternative medicine?

Conventional medicine, at least in recent times, has tended to regard the human body as made up of quite separate parts, each to be treated by a specialist in that part. So, over time, dozens of different medical specialists have developed, each looking at just one part: eyes, ears, throats, skin, mind, and so on. Each separate component is identified, studied, and its particular ways of malfunctioning treated. This approach has been very successful, allowing medical science to overcome most diseases, and its success in many fields is beyond dispute.

But it does not take into account the context in which all the different parts function. Nor does it consider how the owner of these parts thinks, lives, or relates to other people. Could it be that the sort of person you are, the way you live, what you eat, whether you are happily married, and whether you enjoy your job, can affect your state of health?

Conventional medicine can work well if you have a clearly defined disease that fits tidily into one speciality. But with something like irritable bowel syndrome various parts of you are so linked that by rumpling one part (say, your state of mind) you will rumple another (your insides).

This is where you may find a different aproach very helpful. It is known variously as alternative medicine (which, strictly speaking, means it is used instead of conventional medicine), complementary medicine (which means it is used alongside conventional medicine), and holistic medicine (which is a way of looking at the patient as a whole person, and not just as a collection of symptoms). But for the purposes of this book, I use them all interchangeably.

93

The main difference between conventional medicine and alternative medicine is that, whereas the conventional doctor will examine and treat your individual symptoms and you will usually be a passive receiver of whatever treatment is prescribed, the alternative practitioner will look at you in your entirety, as a complete whole person, and you will take an active part in your treatment.

In conventional medicine the patient asks the doctor 'What can *you* do to make me well?' In holistic medicine the patient asks the practitioner 'What can *I* do to make me well?' By taking responsibility for your own health and well-being you will have a greater sense of mastery over your illness.

Until quite recently people did take responsibility for their own health, and assumed that most of the time their bodies were normal and healthy. There were very few drugs available to our ancestors, and these were mainly herbal. Nowadays the pharmaceutical industry is one of the largest and most powerful in the country. Drugs are produced for every possible condition. Whatever our problem, we expect to find a drug to put it right quickly. Instead of asking 'What can I *do* to make myself well?' we probably ask 'What can I *take* to make myself well?' We have lost confidence in our bodies, and their ability to heal themselves.

The advertising power of the drug companies causes us to feel that our bodies are faulty, likely to go wrong, always on the verge of disease, needing attention and treatment from members of the medical profession, aided, of course, by modern drugs. Bear in mind that the over-riding desire of the drugs industry is to sell more drugs.

How often do you see drug advertisements saying that the human body is miraculous? Or that most of us live out our lives without serious disease, or that we can recover from minor ailments (and many serious ones, too) if only we treated our bodies better? We all have a self-healing and self-repair system. Don't ignore it, or override it with drugs. For example, if you eat a normally balanced diet, high in fibre, low in fat, and take moderate exercise, you will not suffer from constipation. If you eat all the wrong foods and take no exercise, you probably will; if, having become constipated, you then come to rely on laxatives, you are overriding your body's normal repair system, until eventually it won't work at all. After all, if you cut your finger, you can watch the process of healing taking place before your very eyes. If such natural healing can take place on the outside of the body where you can see it, surely it can also take place inside where you can't?

Holistic medicine (the word 'holistic' comes from the Greek *holos*, meaning 'whole') works on the basis that disease occurs because the body is out of balance. Too much of this, too little of that; the wrong foods; too much stress; an unhelpful environment, and so on. Correct the balance and the body's own resources will be able to fight disease more effectively. For this reason, all holistic practitioners will aim for a long-term solution by treating the underlying cause, rather than seeking a short-term solution by treating only the symptoms. For unless you can treat the cause, the symptoms will simply keep coming back.

In irritable bowel syndrome anti-spasmodic and anti-depressant drugs will usually work quite well for most people some of the time, just by treating the symptoms. But as IBS can be a long-term condition it is important to find a long-term solution. The fact that there are so many general therapies available is some indication that none of them is totally effective. About one-quarter of people with IBS do not respond well to any form of conventional treatment. (To be fair, perhaps a similar proportion of people do not respond well to alternative therapies either.)

While researching this book, I talked and corresponded with many alternative practitioners, and the majority of them were very optimistic that their particular approach can treat IBS successfully, providing the underlying cause was discovered and tackled. Treatment would probably involve identifying what triggers the IBS; reducing stress; making changes to diet; altering some aspects of lifestyle; and using the alternative approach to get the whole person into a state where the body's energies can work towards recovery. The holistic approach will generally consider IBS as a triangle, each side of which is directly linked to the other two:

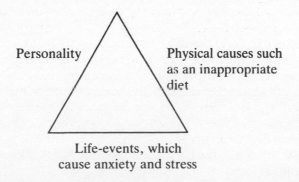

Personality / Physical causes such as an inappropriate diet

Life-events, which cause anxiety and stress

Perhaps you can look at your irritable bowel in this way, and say to yourself 'yes, that makes sense'. Think about how these three aspects link together for you. Then consider what you can do to make changes in each of them. This gentle, non-threatening approach has worked well for many people.

In the next chapter, we will look at some approaches that have a good record of success with IBS. But first a word of caution. As with conventional doctors, alternative therapists do not have all the answers. Be cautious of one who says he has. Some are just as narrow-minded and intolerant of conventional medicine as some conventional doctors are of alternative medicine. Also some believe that their branch of alternative medicine is the only one that will work, and are rather dismissive of any other method. Check the therapist's qualifications (the respected qualifications of each discipline are listed in the next chapter), and if he becomes defensive about his lack of qualifications, go elsewhere.

More and more general practitioners are becoming interested in complementary medicine. Many take training courses, though you should be aware that some of these training courses are very short. Many doctors will also willingly refer patients to alternative practitioners.

If you want to read more widely, your local library probably has a good range of books on alternative medicine. Two which you might consider are *The Handbook of Complementary Medicine*, by Stephen Fuller, published by Coronet in 1984; and *The College of Health Guide to Alternative Medicine*, available from 18 Victoria Park Square, London E2 9PF.

21
How Alternative Medicine Can Help Irritable Bowel Syndrome

'Surely here must be a golden opportunity for practitioners of alternative medicine and devotees of the holistic approach. The traditionalists have not much to boast about.' Letter in *The Lancet*, 1985.

A recent study has suggested that people with IBS are more likely to consult alternative therapists than are other people with gastro-intestinal problems. (Unfortunately, this study did not look further into how successful the different approaches were.) The most favoured therapists are homoeopaths and medical herbalists, but food allergists, hypnotherapists and acupuncturists were also visited. Many herbal and homoeopathic remedies are also bought over the counter for IBS. Usually patients tried these methods when they felt conventional medicine had failed; perhaps they felt the therapist had more time than a busy GP and perhaps they also liked the holistic approach.

Let us now look at how different forms of alternative medicine can help IBS. If you have had it for some time it is unlikely that over-the-counter alternative remedies will have total long-term success. Your problem is probably quite deep-seated, and involves discussion about many aspects of your life with a therapist trained to discover the underlying cause. So you would be well advised to arrange for a personal consultation with a trained practitioner.

How do you know which form of alternative medicine to try? Unfortunately there is no way of knowing which will work best for you. There are many pathways to the same goal. Any therapy (whether conventional or alternative) has a placebo effect, that is, it may work just because you hope it will. But with something as long-term as IBS, in the end you will have to find whatever is right for you.

You can start by asking friends – especially friends with IBS – whether they have had any success with alternative therapies. If your doctor is sympathetic towards alternative medicine, he may recommend someone, although many doctors will only feel able to recommend an alternative practitioner who is also a medically qualified doctor. Choose a therapist either because you have heard well of him or her, or because that form of treatment appeals to you in some way. And keep an open mind about the different approaches. Don't say 'it didn't work for my friend, therefore it won't work for me'. It may.

In many areas of the country several alternative practitioners work from one centre. It will probably be called a Natural Health Clinic, or something similar, and a discussion with the receptionist will give you some idea of which form of help would be right for you.

It is not necessary to know about the philosophy behind any particular branch of alternative medicine for it to work. Nor is it necessary for you to have a firm belief that it will work. After all, many practitioners successfully treat children, and even animals, although these patients can have no expectation of what will happen. You should, however, feel a commitment to allowing it to work, and to using yourself in your own recovery. It would be a rather negative attitude to say 'I am using acupuncture to make me well, so therefore I don't need to do anything for myself'; a more positive and probably successful approach would be to say 'by seeing an acupuncturist I am taking a positive step towards helping myself'.

The forms of alternative medicine which are known to have a good degree of success with IBS are homoeopathy, medical herbalism, osteopathy, hypnotherapy, and acupuncture.

Homoeopathy

Homoeopathy treats 'like with like', that is, the remedy that in a concentrated form brings out a certain reaction in a healthy person –let us say a high fever – will when greatly diluted cure the same or similar symptoms in an unhealthy person. In this respect it is similar to vaccination – introduce a diluted form of, say, diptheria, into the body, and this will enable the body to fight that disease.

Whereas conventional medicine suppresses symptoms, homoeo-pathy regards symptoms as part of the body's attempt to fight disease; therefore symptoms must be respected and not suppressed.

Like most forms of alternative medicine, it is safe, and without side-effects. The results tend to be long-lasting.

Usually, after taking a course of homoeopathic treatment, you will feel very much better in yourself. You will almost certainly experience a greatly increased sense of well-being, and, whether or not your irritable bowel improves rapidly, you will probably feel better able to cope with it. This is a typical response to homoeopathic treatment.

You will be surprised at the questions the homoeopath asks you – what sort of weather do you like, or dislike? Do you prefer rivers or mountains? Do you prefer company or solitude, warm or cold rooms, to take exercise or not? Do you like foods that are sweet or savoury or salty or fatty? What skin problems have you had? Do you express your emotions? What were your parents like? These all give an indication of the sort of person you are. The homoeopath will want to know details of your past medical history, previous operations, general health, and any recurring problems.

After taking all these things into account, he will give you a remedy that is right for your particular constitution and personality. He may or may not give you something specifically for your irritable bowel, and if he does not, that doesn't matter at all. What matters is the whole *you*. After all, he is trying to remove the underlying disturbance which causes the symptoms, rather than treat the symptoms directly.

Homoeopathic tablets need to be taken rather differently from ordinary tablets. Do not handle them – just tip two tablets into the lid of the container, and pop them straight into your mouth without touching them. Suck or chew them, do *not* swallow them whole. Make sure you do not eat or drink anything 20–30 minutes before and after taking the tablets. While taking a course of homoeopathic tablets, avoid all strong flavours, such as coffee, alcohol, cough sweets, mints, and strong toothpaste. Store the tablets away from all strong flavours and smells.

You may notice an improvement quite quickly, or it may take rather longer. As a general guide, reckon that improvement will take about one month for each year that you have had the condition; so that if you have had IBS for, say, four years, it may take about four months to see a great improvement. If there are also deep-seated psychological or other problems, it could take even longer. The homoeopath will probably warn you that your symptoms may get worse before they get better. Surprisingly, this is a good sign, and shows that the remedy is working. If this happens you may be advised to stop taking the remedy just until the symptoms subside. But, be assured that if you follow all the guidance the homoeopath gives you, the results should be long-lasting.

Although IBS will almost certainly require specialist treatment to achieve success, in mild cases that have started quite recently it might be worth trying the following homoeopathic remedies (which are available from many chemists and health-food shops):

Colicky stomach pain

Sharp cramping pains, and warmth gives relief – magnesia phosphorica

If it is eased by firm pressure, or by bending double, if you can't keep still with the pain – colocynthis

If it is eased by stretching backwards or forwards – dioscorea

With 'cutting' pain, and a feeling of nausea with each spasm – ipecacuanha

If it is worse when anticipating any kind of ordeal – argentum nitricum

With much mucus – mercurius solubilis

Constipation

Consider these *in addition to* changes to your diet, more exercise, and a routine that encourages regularity:

When there is a feeling of fullness even after a bowel movement –aesculus or nux vomica.

For stools that are hard to pass – silica

Where over-use of laxatives has caused the bowel muscle to become ineffective – opium (homoeopathic opium, not the sort smoked in opium dens!)

Diarrhoea

With colicky pain, causing you to bend double – colocynthis

Morning diarrhoea, loose and urgent – natrum sulphuricum

Diarrhoea worse after cabbage and other green vegetables – petroleum (the homoeopathic sort, not the kind that goes in cars!)

Distension of abdomen

Wind which is difficult to bring up – carbo vegetabilis

Belching does not make it better – cinchona officinalis

With stomach pain and a feeling of fullness after only a little food –lycopodium

Distension with cramping stomach pain – Magnesia phosphorica

With passing of wind, nausea, and the need to loosen clothing – pulsatilla

With offensive-smelling wind – sulphur

Stomach pain like indigestion

Especially after fatty or oily food – pulsatilla or calcium carbonica

With colicky pain, better for straightening up or bending backwards – dioscerea.

If it is caused by taking lots of indigestion tablets – muriatic acid.

If it is caused by nervous strain, and the pain usually occurs about two hours after eating – nux vomica

If you regurgitate your food, often about one hour after meals – sulphur.

These remedies cover simply the outward symptoms of IBS, and take no account of aspects of your personality and lifestyle which may have contributed to it. Only a qualified homoeopath can decide which 'constitutional' remedy is right for your personality.

It is not easy to recommend what potency of tablets should be taken, or how often. So if you have never taken a homoeopathic remedy before, it would be best if you consulted a qualified homoeopath rather than buying a remedy over the counter.

To find the name of a homoeopath near you, send an s.a.e. to: The Homoeopathic Development Foundation Ltd, 19A Cavendish Square, London W1M 9AD. You can get a list of medically qualified doctors who are also homoeopaths from the British Homoeopathic Association, 27a Devonshire Street, London W1N 1RJ. Look for the qualifications M. F. Hom. or F. F. Hom. (Member, or Fellow of the Faculty of Homoeopathy). For a list of qualified homoeopaths who are not doctors, write to the Society of Homoeopaths, 2a Bedford Place, Southampton SO1 1BY. Look for the qualifications Dip. Hom. (Diploma in Homoeopathy) or R. S. Hom. (Register of the Society of Homoeopaths).

Medical Herbalism

The purpose of herbal remedies is to restore health and introduce a new sense of internal balance. Used correctly, they are without damaging side- effects. Many of today's conventional drugs have their basis in herbal medicine, but because of the way they are manufactured many other qualities are lost.

Plant medicines are most commonly prescribed in liquid form as tinctures, fluid extracts or syrups, but may sometimes be given dried, or as infusions, decoctions, tablets or capsules. They may also be prescribed as ointments, lotions and poultices.

As with conventional medicine, it will be necessary first to exclude any possibility of such conditions as diverticular disease, cancer, ulcerative colitis, Crohn's disease, as well as things like an intolerance to dairy products, or a food allergy.

The aim of the medical herbalist will be to relax the central nervous system so that normal movement of the colon can be achieved without excessive spasm. This will be done with the use of plants which have anti-spasmodic, relaxing, or sedative qualities. Examples of plants which may be chosen are: *Pimpinella anisum* (aniseed); *Mentha piperita* (peppermint); *Matricaria recutita* (camomile); *Lavendula officinalis* (lavender); *Thymus serpyllum* (wild thyme); *Valeriana officinalis* (valerian), and *Stachys betonica* (betony). A bulking agent such as psyllium seeds may be helpful, especially in the diarrhoea form of IBS, to produce a normal bowel movement. The use of demulcent muculagenous plants such as *Althaea radix* (marshmallow root) may also be prescribed.

The medical herbalist will encourage you to develop a lifestyle where you can adapt more successfully to life's stresses and strains.

In contrast with conventional medical practice, you may be advised not to take rough high-residue foods such as nuts and high-fibre cereals, and to try instead root vegetables such as carrots, potatoes, swedes, parsnips, turnips, or various Caribbean or African vegetables.

As with so many forms of alternative medicine, you will be treated as a complete person, mind, body and spirit, and not just as a collection of digestive symptoms. No two people are the same, so each person will receive an individual prescription based on his or her case history and the most appropriate path to health for that person.

Some herbs can be harmful, especially during pregnancy, so make sure the practitioner you consult is properly qualified. Self-help is not recommended. Look for the qualification MNIMH (Member of the National Institute of Medical Herbalists). For a register of practitioners send an s.a.e. to: The National Institute of Medical Herbalists, 41 Hatherley Road, Winchester, Hants.

Osteopathy

Like other holistic approaches to disease, osteopathy tries to find out why the patient has a particular problem at a particular time. It is the reasons behind the disease which influence the osteopath and the way he will treat the patient.

One of the main tenets of osteopathy was laid down in 1870 by Andrew Taylor Still, the founding father of osteopathy. He maintained that *structure governs function*. In other words, if a thing is built correctly and is correctly adjusted and maintained it will do the job it is supposed to do. If, however, it is treated badly and not looked after, then it will break down and fail.

Osteopaths believe that the bones and muscles of the body, and its surrounding nerves and blood vessels, are more than just the framework that support the organs. They believe that these bones and muscles organize good health by a system of reflexes and muscle chains which allow the organs to be correctly suspended within the abdomen, the pelvis and the chest cavity. When this supporting system is overloaded or abused it will fail, and the organs concerned will not work properly. If this continues for too long, abnormalities and disease can occur.

Take, for example, the gut, and especially the large intestine. The function of the large intestine is to collect solid waste matter, and to hold it and store it while water is reabsorbed and minerals are recovered. The passage of this waste matter down the gut is a carefully controlled series of steps allowing digestion to take place in an orderly fashion.

The osteopath, using his knowledge of anatomy and physiology, together with his skill at feeling the tissues and muscles in the spine and abdomen, can diagnose and detect when things are not as they should be.

A series of automatic nerve pathways exist between the organs and the spinal tissues and back again, and by using manipulation and other techniques the osteopath can break into these reflex pathways in an attempt to change or influence anything that is not working properly in the gut. Because IBS is a disorder in which abnormal reflexes lead to the abnormal working of the gut, often caused by stress, the osteopath attempts to treat the condition by using these reflexes themselves.

He also uses the fact that the abdominal organs are enclosed in a muscular 'box', consisting of the pelvic floor below, the diaphragm above, and the abdominal muscles all around. In normal breathing the diaphragm massages the gut from above, and the downward force exerted by the diaphragm is received by the muscles of the pelvic floor. If these muscles are too tight or too loose, perhaps because of stress or after childbirth, then this 'massaging' action does not take place efficiently. Therefore, when treating cases of IBS, the osteopath will want to examine and treat the diaphragm and pelvic floor.

Like other practitioners, the osteopath will emphasize the importance of a suitable diet, especially the inclusion of plenty of fibre, and the development of unhurried toilet habits.

Osteopathy definitely does not lend itself to self-help, and you should ensure the osteopath you visit has a recognized qualification. An inexperienced or unqualified person could do a lot of harm. Look for the qualification D.O. (Diploma in Osteopathy), followed by M.R.O. (Member of the Register of Osteopaths). For a list of qualified osteopaths send £2 and an s.a.e. to: The Register of Osteopaths, 21 Suffolk Street, London SW1Y 4HG. Your local *Yellow Pages* may also have a display advertisement of osteopaths who are members of the General Council and Register of Osteopaths (look under 'Osteopaths'). Be wary of anyone who advertises individually, because the registered osteopath is specifically forbidden by the General Council and Register of Osteopaths to advertise his services.

Hypnotherapy

Hypnotherapy is a form of psychotherapy which uses hypnosis as an aid. It is a far cry from the stage performer who hypnotizes members of the audience for entertainment and amusement.

Hypnotherapy cannot be forced on someone against his will, and the hypnotist has no power over his patient. He cannot extract from you things which you wish to keep secret, nor make you do anything which you do not want to do. Under hypnosis you do not become unconscious, nor do you fall asleep.

Hypnosis simply induces a very pleasant state of relaxation, which is particularly beneficial where symptoms have been induced or made worse by stress. Most people are surprised at how relaxing and pleasant the sensation is. The hypnotist will enable you to draw on inner resources, and be open to suggestions which encourage a new way of looking at life's problems.

He will endeavour to get at the cause of the problem, and help you to resolve it. He does not treat symptoms directly. In the case of IBS, the cause will usually be some form of stress, from home, or work, or leisure activities. He will regard your IBS as due to some disharmony within you, and will work with you to achieve a state of harmony.

As well as working on the stress that makes your IBS worse, he may also spend time suggesting ways in which you can control the intestinal smooth muscle which is going into spasm and causing you pain.

Perhaps he will ask you to place your hand on your abdomen, to imagine that this hand is holding a warm hot water bottle, and learn to relate this sensation of warmth to gaining control over your gut.

To cope with the pain of IBS the hypnotherapist may ask you to form in your mind an image of the pain in whatever way comes most naturally to you – it may be in the form of an animal, or a boa constrictor, or a colour or shape, everyone is different. Then he may ask you to notice the first change that happens as the pain begins to diminish by one-tenth. This technique can be extremely helpful in reducing pain.

The hypnotherapist will show you how to enter an altered state of consciousness called *self-hypnosis*, and then how to use it, by giving you appropriate suggestions to enable you to slow down or speed up the way your bowel is working. The relaxation induced in hypnosis allows your unconscious mind to receive and use suggestions which will be acceptable to you. After learning this technique, you will be able to do it on your own whenever you feel you need it, and will become more and more in control of your bowel. It is important that the suggestions are made to you, and the technique of self-hypnosis taught to you, by a trained hypnotherapist.

Many people with IBS find hypnotherapy extremely beneficial, particularly for stomach pain and distension, and say it increases their feeling of general well-being! Some therapists see patients individually, others use group therapy, and recent research shows both these methods to be equally effective.

There are no medically recognized qualifications in hypnotherapy, and anyone can call himself a hypnotherapist. Medically qualified therapists are not necessarily better, but many people feel more confident if they know the person they see is also a professionally qualified doctor. The two organizations listed below are for those who are already medically qualified. Membership of these organizations is not a qualification, nor are members entitled to use the fact of membership to advertise:

The British Society of Medical and Dental Hypnosis, c/o 42 Links Road, Ashtead, Surrey KT21 2HJ. Look for the initials BSMDH in addition to recognized medical qualifications.

The British Society of Experimental and Clinical Hypnosis, National Secretary: Dr M. Heap, Principal Clinical Psychologist, Department of Psychology, Middlewood Hospital, Sheffield S6 1TP. Look for the initials BSECH.

If you are happy to see a hypnotherapist who is not medically qualified, the following organizations will be able to give you names of hypnotherapists in your area:

The National Council of Psychotherapists and Hypnotherapy Register, 1, Clovelly Road, Ealing, London W5, which maintains a national register of hypnotherapists.

The British Hypnotherapy Association, 67 Upper Berkeley Street, London W1H 7DH. Look for the initials MBHA, ABHA or FBHA – Member, Associate or Fellow of the British Hypnotherapy Association.

National Register of Hypnotherapists and Psychotherapists, 25 Market Square, Nelson, Lancs BB9 7LP. Look for the initials CHP or DHP – Certificate or Diploma in Hypnosis and Psychotherapy.

Acupuncture

Fear not – if you visit an acupuncturist for your IBS you will not end up looking like a pincushion, nor does the procedure bear any resemblance to having an injection.

As with other alternative practitioners, your first consultation will probably last an hour or more. You will be encouraged to talk about what initially triggered your IBS, and to look at what might be causing you anger or anxiety. Chinese medicine has always recognized that emotions can be a cause of physical disease, though this concept has only recently been accepted in Western medicine. Like so much alternative medicine, acupuncture works on the basis of treating the cause, and allowing the cure to occur by itself. The effects of acupuncture are therefore long-lasting, provided you take reasonable care of yourself.

You may be recommended to change to a different diet, adapted to your particular disharmony – avoiding coffee, refined foods, cheese and dairy products, alcohol, spiced foods, and cutting down on meat. If you have wind, cabbage, legumes, peas, beans and brussels sprouts may have to be excluded. As so many people with IBS tend to eat in a hurry, or to eat inadequate meals, you will be encouraged to eat a wholesome nutritious diet, with plenty of greens (such as spinach and cress), rice cakes instead of bread, and to drink half an hour before and after food rather than drinking during a meal.

You may be asked to keep a record of what you eat during the week, together with details of the symptoms particular foods may produce. Once you have discovered what disagrees with you, you will be encouraged to introduce different foods gradually.

For the actual acupuncture treatment, the practitioner will choose about three or four acupuncture points that directly harmonize the colon; most likely these will be on the forearm, feet, legs, abdomen or lower back. The needles are inserted just a few millimetres, and left in place for about 15 minutes. It does not hurt, unless you are so tense that you aggravate it – so, once again, your state of mind influences your healing.

The needles are about the thickness of a hair, and when inserted by a skilled practitioner you will hardly be aware of them. Unused sterile needles are used for each patient, and there should be no bleeding or swelling as the acupuncture points are not situated over blood vessels or vital organs.

You will probably need about three sessions of treatment, together perhaps with a course of Chinese herbal medicine. After that, some people feel a need to return about three times a year to keep their ailment under control. As with homoeopathy, it may take about one month for each year you have had IBS to get a real improvement, so persevere.

As with other forms of alternative medicine, acupuncture will affect the way you feel as a whole person, and will aim to maintain you in a state of health. In ancient China doctors were paid to keep their patients healthy, rather than to treat them when they were sick, and acupuncture was one of the traditional methods of maintaining a state of health.

To find a fully trained and qualified acupuncturist, send an s.a.e. to the Council for Acupuncture, Suite 1, 19a Cavendish Square, London W1M 9AD. The Council has registers of trained and qualified acupuncturists of the following organizations, which are the main professional bodies for practitioners of acupuncture in the United Kingdom:

The British Acupuncture Association (qualification MBAcA), The International Register of Oriental Medicine (qualification MIROM), The Register of Traditional Chinese Medicine (qualification MRTCM), The Traditional Acupuncture Society (qualification MTAcS).

Other forms of alternative medicine

Homoeopathy, herbalism, osteopathy, hypnotherapy and acupuncture are the main forms of alternative medicine for which I know practitioners are optimistic that they can treat IBS with some hope of success. There are, however, many other forms of holistic medicine which are suitable for digestive problems in general.

Reflexology

Reflexology works by applying pressure and massage to the feet. Practitioners believe that there are clearly defined points on the feet which form lines of energy linking with every part of the body. When these pressure points are manipulated, there will be an improvement in the organ to which that pressure point is linked.

A skilled practitioner can tell by massaging the different areas of your feet where in the rest of your body you have problems, because you will feel some discomfort in the area of your foot that relates to the discomforted area of your body.

Although you will probably get most benefit by visiting a practitioner of reflexology, it is possible to do a certain amount yourself, or have someone do it for you.

The success of reflexology may work on the same principle as acupuncture, that is, pressure at the end of a line of energy may release chemicals called endomorphins which reduce pain and can induce a feeling of well-being. It is also possible that by stimulating the nerve endings, the functioning of different organs will benefit.

The sole of the right foot has an area that corresponds to the ascending colon, and the sole of the left foot an area that corresponds to the descending colon (see illustration). The transverse colon that goes across the centre of your abdomen is shared between each foot. The sigmoid colon area runs across the heel area of each foot. If these parts of the feet are carefully massaged, following the direction taken by the contents of the colon (i.e. the digested food) this may cause the whole colon area to improve greatly.

If you would like to try it for yourself, this is what you do. Find a sitting position in which you can comfortably massage the soles of

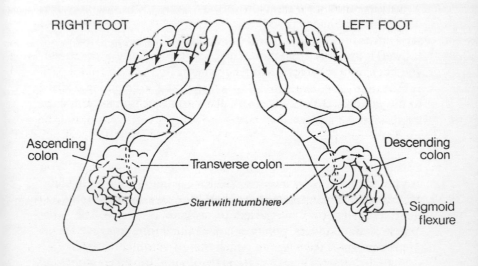

RIGHT FOOT   LEFT FOOT

Ascending colon   Descending colon

Transverse colon

Start with thumb here

Sigmoid flexure

your feet. One possible way is sitting on a chair in such a way that you can place each foot in turn on the thigh of the other leg. Starting with your right foot, place it comfortably on your left thigh (or in any other position that allows easy massage). Place your left thumb in the area shown on the drawing, and massage gently with your thumb up the foot and then across to the edge in the direction of the arrows. As you do this, visualize the corresponding area in your abdomen – up the right side and across the middle. Do this gently several times, always working in the same direction. Then massage the area representing the sigmoid colon, working from the outside of the foot to the inside, as in the drawing.

Now place your left foot comfortably on your right thigh (or wherever else is easiest for you). Bearing in mind that you are attempting to follow the natural direction of the digested food in the colon, place your right thumb on the instep area of the foot, then across to the outside, and down towards the heel in the direction shown on the drawing. Do this gently several times, always working in the same direction. As before, visualize your own colon, from the centre of your abdomen, and down the left side towards the rectum. Then massage the area representing the sigmoid colon, working from the outside of the foot to the inside.

Finally gently massage the underneath of all your toes, working from the top of each toe to the ball of the foot.

As you work on the colon area of your foot, you may feel discomfort, perhaps a prickling feeling, or the sensation of grains of sand under the skin. This is an indication that the area of your colon (bowel) is in need of attention, and by working gently as described, you may see a considerable improvement.

Find time to do these exercises each morning and evening, for five to ten minutes. Take care not to apply too much pressure, which might increase any tension.

Autogenic training

This is an extension of hypnotherapy, but at a self-help level. You can put ideas into your own mind which can help your own healing. Many people feel upset, even insulted, when their doctor tells them their irritable bowel is caused by a state of mind. The label 'psychosomatic illness' conjures up all the wrong images. This is where autogenic training can be particularly useful.

Most doctors will accept that a state of mind can cause a physical illness, and a persistent physical illness can produce an upset state of mind. Now if your mind can affect your body in a harmful way (as with IBS), can you make the mental leap that it can also affect it in a good way? If a poor state of mind can cause IBS, perhaps a good state of mind can improve it. There is proven scientific evidence to show that autogenics can help to reduce high blood pressure and increase mental well-being.

Autogenic training uses the mind to help the body. A sort of 'mind over matter', a cross between self-hypnosis and meditation, it really needs expert tuition, and you cannot easily learn it from books. To find a teacher of autogenic training, send an s.a.e. to: The British Association for Autogenic Training and Therapy, c/o St John's Hospital, Stone, Aylesbury, Bucks. Or to the Positive Health Centre, 101 Harley Street, London W1.

This simple introduction to self-hypnosis may be helpful to you. Relax, following the routine in Chapter 19. Then form a mental picture of anything pleasurable that occurs to you. Hold this in your mind, then let that image change into an image of yourself. Spend time building that image of yourself into someone who has the qualities you desire, such as tranquillity, freedom from stress, freedom from IBS. Then recall a time of your life when you were like this (possibly many years ago, even in childhood), and hold that image. Now project that image of yourself then into an image of yourself today, and hold it. You were like that once, you can be like that again. Finally visualize the 'new' you doing the things you do now, and coping well, and with no irritable bowel syndrome.

Another method is to use an affirmation: Say to yourself 'I have control over my body', and then if you feel this isn't really true, say to yourself 'I haven't, because . . .' Then say again 'I have control over my body', and again 'I haven't because . . .' Continue until you have no further reasons to give. Then say to yourself 'my bowel is quiet and calm, and I can control it'. As you say this try hard to believe it. Place your hands on the area of your ascending and descending colon, feel a sense of warmth and quietness and freedom from spasm.

As self-healing involves a commitment to believing you can be well again, try these visualization exercises:

- Just try to see yourself well again, visualize your IBS being overcome, in any way that makes sense to you.
- Focus on the smooth muscle that propels the digested food, and is the cause of much of the trouble as it goes into spasm. Think

about this area of muscle, visualize it moving in beautiful waves, with warmth, without spasm. Think of the sea, and a sailing boat moving peacefully and gently along on the waves. Transfer this image to the smooth wave-like motion of the muscles of your colon.

● Create in your mind an image of your bowel, in a way that you understand; it doesn't need to be medically accurate – just your own image of your insides. See your colon as a tube of smooth muscle going into painful spasm, the food in it getting held up, forming into pellets, and causing you pain. Then visualize the spasm disappearing, the food in the tube passing in gently rhythmic waves up the right side of your tummy, across the middle and down the left side. See your body making itself well again. If you are on prescribed medicines (anti-spasmodics or bulk laxatives), see them working in your gut. Visualize the effect all this has, giving you normal stools, freedom from pain, freedom to eat whatever you want, quite relaxed. See your irritable bowel as weak, and your body's defences as strong and under your control. Do this exercise two or three times a day. Believe in it. It really does work.

As with all forms of meditation, don't expect instant results. Practise these exercises regularly, and over time you will be surprised at the change in you.

Bach flower remedies

These remedies work by healing the negative states of mind that are thought to be the cause of physical disorders – anger, jealousy, fear, grief, hopelessness, terror, persistent unwanted thoughts, self-distrust, exhaustion, anxiety, irritability, depression, guilt, resentment, bitterness, intolerance, tension, and many others. Perhaps you can see some of your own feelings here, most people can. For further information, send an s.a.e. to: The Edward Bach Centre, Mount Vernon, Sotwell, Wallingford, Oxon OX10 0PZ.

Aromatherapy

Practitioners of aromatherapy administer essential oils to different parts of the body as a form of healing. These oils can help IBS in several ways, both as a direct treatment for the gut, and as a means of controlling stress. The main method is general massage applied by a therapist, and local applications of oil to the abdomen, which you could learn to do for yourself after suitable advice and instruction. You may also be given oils to put in your bath to aid relaxation. In addition, oils may be given as inhalations, tinctures and lotions; they are never taken internally.

To be sure of finding a well-trained therapist, send an s.a.e. to the International Federation of Aromatherapists, 46 Dalkeith Road, London SE21 8LS. Look for the qualification MIFA (Member of the International Federation of Aromatherapists).

If you want to try it yourself, your local health-food or wholefood shop, and some pharmacies, may have stocks of essential oils. It is important to use them correctly, as the wrong use may have the reverse effect, or even provoke an unpleasant reaction. So seek good advice and follow it carefully. There are also several books available, which will guide you on which oils to use, and how to use them. The publishers C. W. Daniel, 1 Church Path, Saffron Walden, Essex, have a good list.

22

In Conclusion

Until recently, IBS was poorly understood, poorly researched, and, to be honest, not of much interest to doctors. But things are changing at last, and a lot of research is going on worldwide.

If your main symptom is painless diarrhoea, if you have had it for only a few months, and if it started after a bout of gastro-enteritis, the outlook is good. Provided you can keep your diet and stress under control you may well be rid of your irritable bowel almost permanently.

If your main IBS symptom is constipation and if you have had it for a few years, you may have to accept that in the present state of medical knowledge a permanent cure still has to be found. But, as I hope you will realize by now, there is a lot you can do to help yourself.

There will be times when it seems to go away completely. When this happens, enjoy these times, and see if you can work out why you haven't got it. If it comes back, don't get depressed about it, just work out what changes you have made in your life, and consider whether you could have done things differently to keep it at bay.

With all the research that is going on into IBS, it is interesting to speculate what the medical profession will come up with in the next few years. They may discover that it is organic, that is, that there is some measurable physical defect in some part of the body. More may be learned about the abnormal motility and overreactivity of the irritable bowel. Disturbances may be discovered in different parts of the gut, and the small intestine may turn out to be as important as the colon and the rectum. Hopefully, simpler ways will be discovered to measure pressure in the colon, and new techniques may make uncomfortable procedures like sigmoidoscopy a thing of the past. With any luck, a simple non-intrusive test will be developed that will enable the doctor to say 'this test is positive, therefore you have irritable bowel syndrome'. And hopefully a treatment will be found that gives long-term improvement, without any side effects.

But until that day comes, your IBS is down to you. It really is one of those conditioins where *you* can make it better or worse.

If you can make some of the changes you have read about in this book, eat a more appropriate diet, try a holistic approach to treatment, view life differently, and above all *relax*, you will have control over your IBS.

So start today. You really *can* make yourself better.

Further Reading

The Food Connection, Colin Tudge, BBC Books 1985
The Allergy Diet, E. Workman, J. Hunter & V. Alun Jones, Martin
   Dunitz 1984
The Food Intolerance Diet Book, E. Workman, V. Alun Jones & J.
   Hunter, Martin Dunitz 1986
Constipation, Piles and other Bowel Disorders, R. Heatley,
   Churchill Livingstone 1984
Medicines—a Guide for Everybody, P. Parish, Penguin 1987
Treating Type 'A' Behaviour and your Heart, M. Friedman and D.
   Ulmer, Michael Joseph 1985
Coping with Stress, Dr Georgia Witkin-Lanoil, Sheldon Press 1985

Medical Books

The following list gives references to more technical books and
medical journals, which provide scientific evidence to back up the
information given here, and which doctors may find useful.

'The irritable colon syndrome' Chaudhary & Truelove, *Q. J. Med*
   1962, *31*, 307
'The irritable bowel—Progress report', *Gut* 1984, *25*, 305
'Towards a positive diagnosis of the irritable bowel', Manning et al.
   BMJ 1978, *3*, 653
'Functional bowel disorders in apparently healthy people',
   Thompson et al. *Gastroenterology* 1980, *79*, 283
Articles in *Stress Management* Supplement of *Den. Clin. North Am.*
   1986, *30*, (4 Suppl)
Dietary Fibre ed. K. Heaton, Libbey 1977
'Functional bowel disease', Heaton, *Rec. Adv. Gastroent* 1988
Irritable Bowel Syndrome, ed. N. W. Read, Grune & Stratton 1985

Index

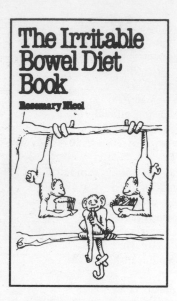

The Irritable
Bowel Diet
Book

Rosemary Nicol

A diet book that will help
you cope with IBS without
disrupting your life. It's
packed with recipes and
suggestions for healthy and
enjoyable meals, and advice
about what to choose for a
snack lunch at work, what
to order in a restaurant and
how to cope when you're
invited out for a meal.

*Available from
all good bookshops,
or direct from*

Sheldon Press Mail Order
36 Steep Hill
Lincoln LN2 1LU
Tel: 0845 762 6747

Also available from Sheldon Press

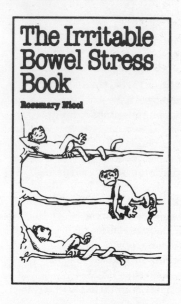

The Irritable
Bowel Stress
Book

Rosemary Nicol

The final piece of the
jigsaw. *The Irritable Bowel
Stress Book* explains how to
handle the stress that can
play such a large part in
causing your IBS. It will
help you understand how
stress, nerves or frustration
can aggravate your IBS and
shows how to combat their
effects, minute by minute in
tense situations, and as part
of everyday life.